# Manual of
# LABORATORY SAFETY

# Manual of
# LABORATORY SAFETY

*(Chemical, Radioactive, and Biosafety with Biocides)*

**Najat Rashid** MSc PhD (UK)
Director
Federal Medical Laboratories
Consultant
Clinical and Molecular Biochemist
Ministry of Health
United Arab Emirates

**Ramnik Sood** MD (Path, Gold Medalist)
Consultant
Reem Medical and Diagnostic Center
Healthcare Mena Limited
Sharjah
United Arab Emirates

*Foreword*
**Mansour Al-Zarouni**

## JAYPEE BROTHERS MEDICAL PUBLISHERS (P) LTD

**New Delhi • London • Philadelphia • Panama**

**Jaypee Brothers Medical Publishers (P) Ltd**

**Headquarters**

Jaypee Brothers Medical Publishers (P) Ltd
4838/24, Ansari Road, Daryaganj
New Delhi 110 002, India
Phone: +91-11-43574357
Fax: +91-11-43574314
**Email: jaypee@jaypeebrothers.com**

**Overseas Offices**

J.P. Medical Ltd
83 Victoria Street, London
SW1H 0HW (UK)
Phone: +44-2031708910
Fax: +02-03-0086180
**Email: info@jpmedpub.com**

Jaypee Medical Inc.
The Bourse
111 South Independence Mall East
Suite 835, Philadelphia, PA 19106, USA
Phone: + 267-519-9789
**Email: joe.rusko@jaypeebrothers.com**

Jaypee Brothers Medical Publishers (P) Ltd
Shorakhute, Kathmandu
Nepal
Phone: +00977-9841528578
**Email: jaypee.nepal@gmail.com**

Jaypee-Highlights Medical Publishers Inc.
City of Knowledge, Bld. 237, Clayton
Panama City, Panama
Phone: + 507-301-0496
Fax: + 507-301-0499
**Email: cservice@jphmedical.com**

Jaypee Brothers Medical Publishers (P) Ltd
17/1-B Babar Road, Block-B, Shaymali
Mohammadpur, Dhaka-1207
Bangladesh
Mobile: +08801912003485
**Email: jaypeedhaka@gmail.com**

Website: www.jaypeebrothers.com
Website: www.jaypeedigital.com

**Inquiries for bulk sales may be solicited at**: jaypee@jaypeebrothers.com

This book has been published in good faith that the contents provided by the authors contained herein are original, and is intended for educational purposes only. While every effort is made to ensure accuracy of information, the publisher and the authors specifically disclaim any damage, liability, or loss incurred, directly or indirectly, from the use or application of any of the contents of this work. If not specifically stated, all figures and tables are courtesy of the authors. Where appropriate, the readers should consult with a specialist or contact the manufacturer of the drug or device.

*Manual of Laboratory Safety*

*First Edition*: **2013**

ISBN : 978-93-5090-622-4

*Printed at:* Ajanta Offset & Packagings Ltd., New Delhi

# Dedicated to

*Our Friend, Philosopher and Guide*

*Dr Ahmed Abdul-Ghaffar Khatib*

# FOREWORD

It gives me immense pleasure to introduce this excellent treatise on safety and security in a medical diagnostic laboratory. Having spent all my working life in such a laboratory, I am well-aware of the problems often encountered in clinical and research laboratories. Although I stood at the apex of the setup, but it was always necessary for me to look down even at the status of the floors of my setup. The tabletops ambient air that we breathed had all to be free from pathogens. I have seen technologists getting Brucellosis by smelling the *Brucella* growing culture plates. Many an individuals have acquired HIV/AIDS from the laboratory and lost their lives (from preventable causes).

This textbook will serve as an ideal partner/companion and tool to make your workplace namely, the laboratory, as the safest place (whether you run a stand-alone laboratory or as part of a hospital setup). A simple step such as keeping the sleeves of your labcoat a little short can prevent spread of methicillin-resistant *Staphylococcus aureus* (MRSA) and fomite transmittable viral diseases.

The measures suggested within the covers of this book are up to date and as per current internationally acceptable standards and protocols. What World Health Organization (WHO) recommends, what Centers for Disease Control (CDC) recommends—the reader will find everything just by flipping a few pages.

**Mansour Al-Zarouni** BSc (USA), MSc and PhD (UK)
Consultant
Medical and Molecular Microbiologist
Head
Department of Pathology and Laboratory Medicine
Sharjah Medical District
Ministry of Health
United Arab Emirates

# PREFACE

Medical diagnostic laboratories can usually be classified into basic or primary, medium or secondary, and advanced or tertiary laboratories. However, one fact cannot be overlooked that they are and can be the most dangerous places in a hospital for the personnel working in them and for individuals who visit them. Most cases or samples that reach a laboratory come with a presumption that they are pathological or abnormal. Consequently, one has to exercise more precautions in a laboratory as compared to other regions of a healthcare providing facility. Needless to say that the basic or peripherally situated laboratories would normally have the least protective measures in place. Also, one has to remember that besides harboring bacteria, viruses; all laboratories also house numerous simple and dangerous chemicals and some even deal with radioactive materials and substances. So, all laboratories must have all provisions and adequately understand the concepts and designs and operations/ methods to keep a laboratory safe at all times for all those who visit them either as workers or as patients. One could pick up MRSA or H1N1 virus from the tabletop. One could easily carry them home and put others at risk—individuals who have nothing to do with medical diagnostic laboratory. While working in a laboratory there may be a spill sometime, so everyone must know how to deal with them. Personal accidents can and do happen. One must, as a matter of principle, avoid working alone in a laboratory at all times. The person not involved in the accident in the laboratory comes in handy in saving the life of the other.

Also with the emergence of rules that make laboratories mandatorily to be International Organization for Standardization (ISO)/Joint Commission International (JCI) or Certified Authorization Professional (CAP) certified or compliant, the laboratory safety measures acquire greater significance. Without perfect safety measures in place, such accreditations are never granted.

So, peep within the pages of this book and get "A to Z" of all aspects related to laboratory safety and security. The book amply covers biosafety and biosecurity while not forgetting safety with chemicals and radioactive materials. The book suggests measures to prevent accidents and should they happen, what to do under those circumstances.

Why wait, own this copy and take it to your place and start checklisting the appropriate measures that you have and those that you do not have. Set them right and make your facility as safe if possible and necessary.

We would like to place on record the help and assistance rendered by Mr Abdul Razaq Donigal Mohammed, without his unceasing passion, this book would not have seen the light of the day.

**Najat Rashid**
**Ramnik Sood**

# CONTENTS

**CHAPTER FIVE**

# Chapter One

# Biosafety

## INTRODUCTION

The purpose of this manual is to be a resource for information, guidelines, policies, and procedures that will enable and encourage those working in the laboratory environment to work safely and reduce or eliminate the potential for exposure to biological, chemical and radioactive materials hazard.

The goal of the laboratory safety is to minimize the risk of injury and illness to laboratory workers by ensuring they have the training, information, support and equipment needed.

The manual promotes safe and practical laboratory procedures, included laboratory biosafety, laboratory biosecurity, microbiological risk assessment, laboratory biosafety levels, information on the use of personal protective equipment, laboratory animal facilities, laboratories equipment, laboratory techniques, hazard communication and packing of infectious substances, biosafety and biotechnology, the proper use of disinfection and sterilization, the use and storage of chemicals and radioactive materials, biosafety officer and biosafety committee and the proper methods of waste disposal.

Finally, emphasis must be placed on the practices and procedures used by trained laboratory staff. Since "no biosafety cabinet or other facility or procedure alone guarantees safety unless the users operate safe techniques based on informed understanding." It is the responsibility of everyone, including managers and laboratory workers, to use the information available in these manual and to perform their work in a safe and secure manner.

## LABORATORY BIOSAFETY

'Laboratory biosafety' is the term used to describe the containment principles, technologies and practices that are implemented to prevent unintentional exposure to pathogens and toxins, or their accidental release.

A laboratory biosafety goal is to ensure that hazardous materials will be handled and disposed of in such a way that people, other living organisms, and the environment are protected from harm. Safety awareness must be a part of everyone's habits, and can only be achieved if all senior and responsible staff has a sincere, visible, and continuing interest in preventing injuries and occupational illnesses.

Laboratory facilities are designated as: Basic Biosafety Level 1 (BSL-1), Basic Biosafety Level 2 (BSL-2), Containment Biosafety Level 3 (BSL-3) and Maximum containment Biosafety Level 4 (BSL-4).

## Biosafety Level 1

Practices, safety equipment, and facility design and construction are appropriate for undergraduate and secondary educational training and teaching laboratories, and for other laboratories in which work is done with defined and characterized strains of viable microorganisms not known to consistently cause disease in healthy adult humans. *Bacillus subtilis, Naegleria gruberi*, infectious canine hepatitis virus, and exempt organisms.

BSL-1 represents a basic level of containment that relies on standard microbiological practices with no special primary or secondary barriers recommended, other than a sink for handwashing.

## Biosafety Level 2

Practices, equipment, and facility design and construction are applicable to clinical, diagnostic, teaching, and other laboratories in which work is done with the broad spectrum of indigenous moderate-risk agents that are present in the community and associated with human disease of varying severity. With good microbiological techniques, these agents can be used safely in activities conducted on the open bench, provided the potential for producing splashes or aerosols is low. Hepatitis B virus, HIV, the *Salmonella*, and *Toxoplasma* are representative of microorganisms to this containment level. BSL-2 is appropriate when work is done with any human-derived blood, body fluids, tissues, or primary human cell lines where the presence of an infectious agent may be unknown.

- Primary hazards to personnel working with these agents relate to accidental percutaneous or mucous membrane exposures, or ingestion of infectious materials. Extreme caution should be taken with contaminated needles or sharp instruments. Even though organisms routinely manipulated at BSL-2 are not known to be transmissible by the aerosol route, procedures with aerosol or high splash potential that may increase the risk of such personnel exposure must be conducted in primary containment equipment, or in devices such as a BSC or safety centrifuge cups. Personal protective equipment should be used as appropriate, such as splash shields, face protection, gowns, and gloves.
- Secondary barriers, such as hand washing sinks and waste decontamination facilities, must be available to reduce potential environmental contamination.

## Biosafety Level 3

Practices, safety equipment, and facility design and construction are applicable to clinical, diagnostic, teaching, research, or production facilities in which work is done with indigenous or exotic agents with a potential for respiratory transmission, and which may cause serious and potentially lethal infection. *Mycobacterium tuberculosis*, St. Louis encephalitis virus, and *Coxiella burnetii* are representative of the microorganisms assigned to this level. Primary hazards to personnel working with these agents relate to autoinoculation, ingestion, and exposure to infectious aerosols. At BSL-3, more emphasis is placed on:

- Primary barriers to protect personnel in contiguous areas, the community, and the environment from exposure to potentially infectious aerosols. For example, all laboratory manipulations should be performed in a BSC or other enclosed equipment, such as a gas-tight aerosol generation chamber.
- Secondary barriers for this level include controlled access to the laboratory and ventilation requirements that minimize the release of infectious aerosols from the laboratory.

## Biosafety Level 4

Practices, safety equipment, and facility design and construction are applicable for work with dangerous and exotic agents that pose a high individual risk of life-threatening disease, which may be transmitted via the aerosol route and for which there is no available vaccine or therapy. Agents with a close or identical antigenic relationship to BSL-4 agents also should be handled at this level. When sufficient data are obtained, work with these agents may continue at this level or at a lower level. Viruses such as Marburg or Congo-Crimean hemorrhagic fever are manipulated at BSL-4.

Biosafety level designations are based on a composite of the design features, construction, containment facilities, equipment, practices and operational procedures required for working with agents from the various risk groups. The primary hazards to personnel working with BSL-4 agents are respiratory exposure to infectious aerosols, mucous membrane or broken skin exposure to infectious droplets, and autoinoculation. All manipulations of potentially infectious diagnostic materials, isolates, and naturally or experimentally infected animals, pose a high-risk of exposure and infection to laboratory personnel, the community, and the environment.

The assignment of an agent to a biosafety level for laboratory work must be based on a risk assessment. Such an assessment will take the risk group as well as other factors into consideration in establishing the appropriate biosafety level. For example, an agent that is assigned to Risk Group 2 may generally require Biosafety Level 2 facilities, equipment, practices and procedures for safe conduct of work. However, if particular experiments require the generation of high-concentration aerosols, then Biosafety Level 3 may be more appropriate to provide the necessary degree of safety, since it ensures superior containment of aerosols in the laboratory workplace. The biosafety level assigned for the specific work to be done is therefore driven by professional judgment based on a risk assessment, rather than by automatic assignment of a laboratory biosafety level according to the particular risk group designation of the pathogenic agent to be used.

Classification of infective microorganisms by risk group:
- **Risk Group 1 (no or low individual and community risk):** A microorganism that is unlikely to cause human or animal disease.
- **Risk Group 2 (moderate individual risk, low community risk):** A pathogen that can cause human or animal disease but is unlikely to be a serious hazard to laboratory workers, the community, livestock or the environment. Laboratory exposures may cause serious infection, but effective treatment and preventive measures are available and the risk of spread of infection is limited.

- **Risk Group 3 (high individual risk, low community risk):** A pathogen that usually causes serious human or animal disease but does not ordinarily spread from one infected individual to another. Effective treatment and preventive measures are available.
- **Risk Group 4 (high individual and community risk):** A pathogen that usually causes serious human or animal disease and that can be readily transmitted from one individual to another, directly or indirectly. Effective treatment and preventive measures are not usually available.

Effective biosafety practices are the very foundation of "laboratory biosecurity" activities.

In the absence of careful implementation, various aspects of biosafety may conflict with laboratory biosecurity. For example, controls that reduce unauthorized access might also hinder an emergency response by fire or rescue personnel. Mechanisms need to be established that allow entry by emergency responders but ensure uninterrupted and constant laboratory biosecurity, control and accountability.

Signage may also represent a potential conflict between biosafety and laboratory biosecurity. In the past, biohazard signs placed on laboratory doors identified the biological agents present in the laboratory. However, as a laboratory biosecurity measure to better protection it is recommended certain information on biohazard signs to the laboratory biosafety level, the name and telephone number of the responsible investigator, and emergency contact information (Table 1.1).

## MICROBIOLOGICAL RISK-ASSESSMENT

The backbone of the practice of biosafety is risk-assessment. While there are many tools available to assist in the assessment of risk for a given procedure or experiment, the most important component is professional judgment. Risk assessments should be performed by the individuals most familiar with the specific characteristics of the organisms being considered for use, the equipment and procedures to be employed, animal models that may be used, and the containment equipment and facilities available. The laboratory director or principal investigator is responsible for ensuring that adequate and timely risk assessments are performed, and for working closely with the institution's safety committee and biosafety personnel to ensure that appropriate equipment and facilities are available to support the work being considered. Once performed, risk assessments should be reviewed routinely and revised when necessary, taking into consideration the acquisition of new data having a bearing on the degree of risk and other relevant new information from the scientific literature. One of the most helpful tools available for performing a microbiological risk assessment is the listing of risk groups for microbiological agents. However, simple reference to the risk grouping for a particular agent is insufficient in the conduct of a risk assessment. Other factors that should be considered, as appropriate, include:

1. Pathogenicity of the agent and infectious dose.
2. Natural route of infection.
3. Other routes of infection, resulting from laboratory manipulations (parenteral, airborne, ingestion).
5. Stability of the agent in the environment.

■ **Table 1.1** Biosafety level requirements

| | Biosafety level | | | |
|---|---|---|---|---|
| | 1 | 2 | 3 | 4 |
| Isolation[a] of laboratory | No | No | Yes | Yes |
| Room sealable for decontamination | No | No | Yes | Yes |
| Ventilation: | | | | |
| — Inward airflow | No | Desirable | Yes | Yes |
| — Controlled ventilating system | No | Desirable | Yes | Yes |
| — HEPA-filtered air exhaust | No | No | Yes/No[b] | Yes |
| Double-door entry | No | No | Yes | Yes |
| Airlock | No | No | No | Yes |
| Airlock with shower | No | No | No | Yes |
| Anteroom | No | No | Yes | — |
| Anteroom with shower | No | No | Yes/No[c] | No |
| Effluent treatment | No | No | Yes/No[c] | Yes |
| Autoclave: | | | | |
| — On site | No | Desirable | Yes | Yes |
| — In laboratory room | No | No | Desirable | Yes |
| — Double-ended | No | No | Desirable | Yes |
| Biological safety cabinets | No | Desirable | Yes | Yes |
| Personnel safety monitoring capability[d] | No | No | Desirable | Yes |

[a] Environmental and functional isolation from general traffic
[b] Dependent on location of exhaust
[c] Dependent on agent(s) used in the laboratory
[d] For example, window, closed-circuit television, two-way communication

6. Concentration of the agent and volume of concentrated material to be manipulated.
7. Presence of a suitable host (human or animal).
8. Information available from animal studies and reports of laboratory-acquired infections or clinical reports.
9. Laboratory activity planned for example (sonication, aerosolization, centrifugation, etc.).
10. Any genetic manipulation of the organism that may extend the host range of the agent or alter the agent's sensitivity to known, effective treatment regimens.
11. Local availability of effective prophylaxis or therapeutic interventions.

On the basis of the information ascertained during the risk assessment, a biosafety level can be assigned to the planned work, appropriate personal protective equipment selected, and standard operating procedures (SOPs) incorporating other safety interventions developed to ensure the safest possible conduct of the work.

### Specimens for which there is Limited Information

The risk assessment procedure described above works well when there is adequate information available. However, there are situations when the information is insufficient to perform an appropriate risk assessment, for example, with clinical specimens or epidemiological samples collected in the field. In these cases, it is prudent to take a cautious approach to specimen manipulation.

1. Standard precautions should always be followed, and barrier protections applied (gloves, gowns, eye protection), whenever samples are obtained from patients.
2. Basic containment, Biosafety Level 2 practices and procedures should be the minimum requirement for handling specimens.
3. Transport of specimens should follow national and/or international rules and regulations.

### Some Information may be Available to Assist in Determining the Risk of Handling these Specimens

1. Medical data on the patient.
2. Epidemiological data (morbidity and mortality data, suspected route of transmission, other outbreak investigation data).
3. Information on the geographical origin of the specimen.

### Emergency Procedures in Microbiological Laboratories

#### Puncture Wounds, Cuts and Abrasions

The affected individual should remove protective clothing, wash the hands and any affected area(s), apply an appropriate skin disinfectant, and seek medical attention as necessary. The cause of the wound and the organisms involved should be reported, and appropriate and complete medical records kept.

#### Ingestion of Potentially Infectious Material

Protective clothing should be removed and medical attention sought. Identification of the material ingested and circumstances of the incident should be reported, and appropriate and complete medical records kept.

#### Potentially Infectious Aerosol Release (Outside a Biological Safety Cabinet)

All persons should immediately vacate the affected area and any exposed persons should be referred for medical advice. The laboratory supervisor and the biosafety officer should be informed at once. No one should enter the room for an appropriate amount of time (e.g. 1 h), to allow aerosols to be carried away and heavier particles to settle. If the laboratory does not have a central air exhaust system, entrance should be delayed (e.g. for 24 h).

Signs should be posted indicating that entry is forbidden. After the appropriate time, decontamination should proceed, supervised by the biosafety officer. Appropriate protective clothing and respiratory protection should be worn.

### Broken Containers and Spilled Infectious Substances

Broken containers contaminated with infectious substances and spilled infectious substances should be covered with a cloth or paper towels. Disinfectant should then be poured over these and left for the appropriate amount of time. The cloth or paper towels and the broken material can then be cleared away; glass fragments should be handled with forceps. The contaminated area should then be swabbed with disinfectant. If dustpans are used to clear away the broken material, they should be autoclaved or placed in an effective disinfectant. Cloths, paper towels and swabs used for cleaning up should be placed in a contaminated-waste container. Gloves should be worn for all these procedures.

### Breakage of Tubes Containing Potentially Infectious Material in Centrifuges not having Sealable Buckets

If a breakage occurs or is suspected while the machine is running, the motor should be switched off and the machine left closed (e.g. for 30 minutes) to allow settling. If a breakage is discovered after the machine has stopped, the lid should be replaced immediately and left closed (e.g. for 30 minutes). In both instances, the biosafety officer should be informed.

Strong (e.g. thick rubber) gloves, covered if necessary with suitable disposable gloves, should be worn for all subsequent operations. Forceps, or cotton held in the forceps, should be used to retrieve glass debris.

All broken tubes, glass fragments, buckets, and the rotor should be placed in a noncorrosive disinfectant known to be active against the organisms concerned). Unbroken, capped tubes may be placed in disinfectant in a separate container and recovered.

The centrifuge bowl should be swabbed with the same disinfectant, at the appropriate dilution, and then swabbed again, washed with water and dried. All materials used in the clean-up should be treated as infectious waste.

### Breakage of Tubes Inside Sealable Buckets (Safety Cups)

All sealed centrifuge buckets should be loaded and unloaded in a biological safety cabinet. If breakage is suspected within the safety cup, the safety cap should be loosened the bucket autoclaved. Alternatively, the safety cup may be chemically disinfected.

## LABORATORIES BIOSAFETY LEVELS

For the purposes of this manual, the guidance and recommendations given as minimum requirements pertaining to laboratories of all biosafety levels are directed at microorganisms in Risk Groups 1–4. Although some of the precautions may appear to be unnecessary for some organisms in Risk Group 1, they are desirable for training purposes to promote good (i.e. safe) microbiological techniques GMT. Diagnostic and health-care laboratories (public health, clinical or hospital-based) must all be designed for Biosafety Level 2 or above. As no laboratory has complete control over the specimens it receives, laboratory workers may be exposed to organisms in higher risk groups than anticipated. This possibility must be recognized in the development of safety plans and policies. In some countries, accreditation of clinical laboratories is required. Globally, standard precautions should always be adopted and practiced.

The guidelines for basic laboratories, Biosafety Levels 1 and 2 presented here are comprehensive and detailed, as they are fundamental to laboratories of all biosafety levels. The guidelines for containment laboratories, Biosafety Level 3 and maximum containment laboratories, Biosafety Level 4 are modifications of and additions to these guidelines, designed for work with the more dangerous (hazardous) pathogens.

## Code of Practice

This code is a listing of the most essential laboratory practices and procedures that are basic to GMT. In many laboratories and national laboratory programs, this code may be used to develop written practices and procedures for safe laboratory operations. Each laboratory should adopt a safety or operations manual that identifies known and potential hazards, and specifies practices and procedures to eliminate or minimize such hazards. GMT is fundamental to laboratory safety. Specialized laboratory equipment is a supplement to but can never replace appropriate procedures. The most important concepts are listed below:

### Access

1. The international biohazard warning symbol and sign must be displayed on the doors of the rooms where microorganisms of Risk Group 2 or higher risk groups are handled (Figure 1.1).
2. Only authorized persons should be allowed to enter the laboratory working areas.
3. Laboratory doors should be kept closed.
4. Children should not be authorized or allowed to enter laboratory working areas.
5. Access to animal houses should be specially authorized.
6. No animals should be admitted other than those involved in the work of the laboratory.

### Personal Protection

1. Laboratory coveralls, gowns or uniforms must be worn at all times for work in the laboratory.
2. Appropriate gloves must be worn for all procedures that may involve direct or accidental contact with blood, body fluids and other potentially infectious materials or infected animals. After use, gloves should be removed aseptically and hands must then be washed.
3. Personnel must wash their hands after handling infectious materials and animals, and before they leave the laboratory working areas.
4. Safety glasses, face shields (visors) or other protective devices must be worn when it is necessary to protect the eyes and face from splashes, impacting objects and sources of artificial ultraviolet radiation.
5. It is prohibited to wear protective laboratory clothing outside the laboratory, e.g. in canteens, coffee rooms, offices, libraries, staff rooms and toilets.

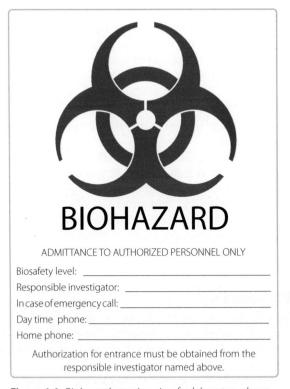

**Figure 1.1** Biohazard warning sign for laboratory doors

6.  Open-toed footwear must not be worn in laboratories.
7.  Eating, drinking, smoking, applying cosmetics and handling contact lenses is prohibited in the laboratory working areas.
8.  Storing human foods or drinks anywhere in the laboratory working areas is prohibited.
9.  Protective laboratory clothing that has been used in the laboratory must not be stored in the same lockers or cupboards as street clothing.

## *Procedures*

1.  Pipetting by mouth must be strictly forbidden.
2.  Materials must not be placed in the mouth. Labels must not be licked.
3.  All technical procedures should be performed in a way that minimizes the formation of aerosols and droplets.
4.  The use of hypodermic needles and syringes should be limited. They must not be used as substitutes for pipetting devices or for any purpose other than parenteral injection or aspiration of fluids from laboratory animals.
5.  All spills, accidents and overt or potential exposures to infectious materials must be reported to the laboratory supervisor. A written record of such accidents and incidents should be maintained.
6.  A written procedure for the clean-up of all spills must be developed and followed.

7.  Contaminated liquids must be decontaminated (chemically or physically) before discharge to the sanitary sewer. An effluent treatment system may be required, depending on the risk assessment for the agent(s) being handled.
8.  Written documents that are expected to be removed from the laboratory need to be protected from contamination while in the laboratory.

## Laboratory Working Areas

1.  The laboratory should be kept neat, clean and free of materials that are not pertinent to the work.
2.  Work surfaces must be decontaminated after any spill of potentially dangerous material and at the end of the working day.
3.  All contaminated materials, specimens and cultures must be decontaminated before disposal or cleaning for reuse.
4.  Packing and transportation must follow applicable national and/or international regulations.
5.  When windows can be opened, they should be fitted with arthropod-proof screens.

## Biosafety Management

1.  It is the responsibility of the laboratory director (the person who has immediate responsibility for the laboratory) to ensure the development and adoption of a biosafety management plan and a safety or operations manual.
2.  The laboratory supervisor (reporting to the laboratory director) should ensure that regular training in laboratory safety is provided.
3.  Personnel should be advised of special hazards, and required to read the safety or operations manual and follow standard practices and procedures. The laboratory supervisor should make sure that all personnel understand these. A copy of the safety or operations manual should be available in the laboratory.
4.  There should be an arthropod and rodent control program.
5.  Appropriate medical evaluation, surveillance and treatment should be provided for all personnel in case of need, and adequate medical records should be maintained.

## Laboratory Design and Facilities

In designing a laboratory and assigning certain types of work to it, special attention should be paid to conditions that are known to pose safety problems. These include:

1.  Formation of aerosols.
2.  Work with large volumes and/or high concentrations of microorganisms.
3.  Overcrowding and too much equipment.
4.  Infestation with rodents and arthropods.
5.  Unauthorized entrance.
6.  Workflow: Use of specific samples and reagents.

## Laboratory Equipment

Together with good procedures and practices, the use of safety equipment will help to reduce risks when dealing with biosafety hazards. This section deals with basic principles related to equipment suitable for laboratories of all biosafety levels.

The laboratory director should, after consultation with the biosafety officer and safety committee (if designated), ensure that adequate equipment is provided and that it is used properly. Equipment should be selected to take account of certain general principles, i.e. it should be:

1. Designed to prevent or limit contact between the operator and the infectious material.
2. Constructed of materials that are impermeable to liquids, resistant to corrosion and meet structural requirements.
3. Fabricated to be free of burrs, sharp edges and unguarded moving parts.
4. Designed, constructed and installed to facilitate simple operation and provide for ease of maintenance, cleaning, decontamination and certification testing. Glassware and other breakable materials should be avoided, whenever possible.

## Essential Biosafety Equipment

1. Pipetting aids, to avoid mouth pipetting. Many different designs are available.
2. Biological safety cabinets, to be used whenever:
   - Infectious materials are handled. Such materials may be centrifuged in the open laboratory if sealed centrifuge safety cups are used and if they are loaded and unloaded in a biological safety cabinet there is an increased risk of airborne infection.
   - Procedures with a high potential for producing aerosols are used. These may include centrifugation, grinding, blending, vigorous shaking or mixing, sonic disruption, opening of containers of infectious materials (whose internal pressure may be different from the ambient pressure), intranasal inoculation of animals, and harvesting of infectious tissues from animals and eggs.
3. Plastic disposable transfer loops. Alternatively, electric transfer loop incinerators may be used inside the biological safety cabinet to reduce aerosol production.
4. Screw-capped tubes and bottles.
5. Autoclaves or other appropriate means to decontaminate infectious materials.
6. Plastic disposable Pasteur pipettes, whenever available, to avoid glass.
7. Equipment such as autoclaves and biological safety cabinets must be validated with appropriate methods before being taken into use.

## Guidelines for the Surveillance of Laboratory Workers Handling Microorganisms at Biosafety Level 1

Historical evidence indicates that the microorganisms handled at this level are unlikely to cause human disease or animal disease of veterinary importance. Ideally, however, all laboratory workers should undergo a pre-employment health check at which their medical history is recorded. Prompt reporting of illnesses or laboratory accidents is desirable and all staff members should be made aware of the importance of maintaining GMT.

### *Guidelines for the Surveillance of Laboratory Workers Handling Microorganisms at Biosafety Level 2*

1. A pre-employment or preplacement health check is necessary. The person's medical history should be recorded and a targeted occupational health assessment performed.
2. Records of illness and absence should be kept by the laboratory management.
3. Women of childbearing age should be made aware of the risk to an unborn child of occupational exposure to certain microorganisms, e.g. rubella virus. The precise steps taken to protect the fetus will vary, depending on the microorganisms to which the women may be exposed.

## Training

Human error and poor technique can compromise the best of safeguards to protect the laboratory worker. Thus, a safety conscious staff, well-informed about the recognition and control of laboratory hazards, is key to the prevention of laboratory acquired infections, incidents and accidents. For this reason, continuous in-service training in safety measures is essential. An effective safety program begins with the laboratory managers, who should ensure that safe laboratory practices and procedures are integrated into the basic training of employees. Training in safety measures should be an integral part of new employees' introduction to the laboratory. Employees should be introduced to the code of practice and to local guidelines, including the safety or operations manual. Measures to assure that employees have read and understood the guidelines, such as signature pages, should be adopted. Laboratory supervisors play the key role in training their immediate staff in good laboratory techniques. The biosafety officer can assist in training and with the development of training aids and documentation.

Staff training should always include information on safe methods for highly hazardous procedures that are commonly encountered by all laboratory personnel and which involve:

1. Inhalation risks (i.e. aerosol production) when using loops, streaking agar plates, pipetting, making smears, opening cultures, taking blood/serum samples, centrifuging, etc.
2. Ingestion risks when handling specimens, smears and cultures.
3. Risks of percutaneous exposures when using syringes and needles.
4. Bites and scratches when handling animals.
5. Handling of blood and other potentially hazardous pathological materials.
6. Decontamination and disposal of infectious material.

## Waste Handling

Waste is anything that is to be discarded. In laboratories, decontamination of wastes and their ultimate disposal are closely interrelated. In terms of daily use, few if any contaminated materials will require actual removal from the laboratory or destruction. Most glassware, instruments and laboratory or clothing will be reused or recycled.

The overriding principle is that all infectious materials should be decontaminated, autoclaved or incinerated within the laboratory.

The principal questions to be asked before discharge of any objects or materials from laboratories that deal with potentially infectious microorganisms or animal tissues are:

1. Have the objects or materials been effectively decontaminated or disinfected by an approved procedure?
2. If not, have they been packaged in an approved manner for immediate on-site incineration or transfer to another facility with incineration capacity?
3. Does the disposal of the decontaminated objects or materials involve any additional potential hazards, biological or otherwise, to those who carry out the immediate disposal procedures or who might come into contact with discarded items outside the facility?

## Decontamination

Steam autoclaving is the preferred method for all decontamination processes. Materials for decontamination and disposal should be placed in containers, e.g. autoclavable plastic bags, that are color-coded according to whether the contents are to be autoclaved and/or incinerated. Alternative methods may be envisaged only if they remove and/or kill microorganisms.

## Handling and Disposal Procedures for Contaminated Materials and Wastes

Identification and separation system for infectious materials and their containers should be adopted. National and international regulations must be followed. Categories should include:

1. Non-contaminated (non-infectious) waste that can be reused or recycled or disposed of as general, "household" waste.
2. Contaminated (infectious) "sharps"—hypodermic needles, scalpels, knives and broken glass; these should always be collected in puncture proof containers fitted with covers and treated as infectious.
3. Contaminated material for decontamination by autoclaving and thereafter washing and reuse or recycling.
4. Contaminated material for autoclaving and disposal.
5. Contaminated material for direct incineration.

## Sharps

After use, hypodermic needles should not be recapped, clipped or removed from disposable syringes. The complete assembly should be placed in a sharps disposal container.

Disposable syringes, used alone or with needles, should be placed in sharps disposal containers and incinerated, with prior autoclaving if required.

Sharps disposal containers must be puncture-proof/resistant and must not be filled to capacity. When they are three-quarters full they should be placed in "infectious waste" containers and incinerated, with prior autoclaving if laboratory practice requires it. Sharps disposal containers must not be discarded in landfills.

### Contaminated Materials for Autoclaving and Reuse

No precleaning should be attempted of any contaminated materials to be autoclaved and reused. Any necessary cleaning or repair must be done only after autoclaving or disinfection.

### Contaminated Materials for Disposal

Apart from sharps, which are dealt with above, all contaminated materials should be autoclaved in leak proof containers, e.g. autoclavable, color-coded plastic bags, before disposal.

After autoclaving, the material may be placed in transfer containers for transport to the incinerator. If possible, materials deriving from health care activities should not be discarded in landfills even after decontamination. If an incinerator is available on the laboratory site, autoclaving may be omitted. The contaminated waste should be placed in designated containers (e.g. color coded bags) and transported directly to the incinerator. Reusable transfer containers should be leak proof and have tight-fitting covers. They should be disinfected and cleaned before they are returned to the laboratory for further use.

Discard containers, pans or jars, preferably unbreakable (e.g. plastic), should be placed at every work station. When disinfectants are used, waste materials should remain in intimate contact with the disinfectant (i.e. not protected by air bubbles) for the appropriate time, according to the disinfectant used. The discard containers should be decontaminated and washed before reuse. Incineration of contaminated waste must meet with the approval of the public health and air pollution authorities, as well as that of the laboratory biosafety officer.

### Biosafety Level 3 (The Containment Laboratory)

The containment laboratory, Biosafety Level 3 is designed and provided for work with Risk Group 3 microorganisms and with large volumes or high concentrations of Risk Group 2 microorganisms that pose an increased risk of aerosol spread. Biosafety Level 3 containment requires the strengthening of the operational and safety program over and above those for basic laboratories, Biosafety Levels 1 and 2.

The guidelines given in this chapter are presented in the form of additions to those for basic laboratories, Biosafety Levels 1 and 2, which must therefore be applied before those specific for the containment laboratory, Biosafety Level 3.

### The Major Additions and Changes

1. Code of practice
2. Laboratory design and facilities
3. Health and medical surveillance.

Laboratories in this category should be registered or listed with the national or other appropriate health authorities.

### Code of Practice

The code of practice for basic laboratories, Biosafety Levels 1 and 2 applies except where modified as follows:

1.  The international biohazard warning symbol and sign displayed on laboratory access doors must identify the biosafety level and the name of the laboratory supervisor who controls access, and indicate any special conditions for entry into the area, e.g. immunization.
2.  Laboratory protective clothing must be of the type with solid-front or wrap-around gowns, scrub suits, coveralls, head covering and, where appropriate, shoe covers or dedicated shoes. Front-buttoned standard laboratory coats are unsuitable, as are sleeves that do not fully cover the forearms. Laboratory protective clothing must not be worn outside the laboratory, and it must be decontaminated before it is laundered. The removal of street clothing and change into dedicated laboratory clothing may be warranted when working with certain agents (e.g. agricultural or zoonotic agents).
3.  Open manipulations of all potentially infectious material must be conducted within a biological safety cabinet or other primary containment device.
4.  Respiratory protective equipment may be necessary for some laboratory Procedures or working with animals infected with certain pathogens.

## Laboratory Design and Facilities

The laboratory design and facilities for basic laboratories—Biosafety Levels 1 and 2 apply except where modified as follows:

1.  The laboratory must be separated from the areas that are open to unrestricted traffic flow within the building. Additional separation may be achieved by placing the laboratory at the blind end of a corridor, or constructing a partition and door or access through an anteroom (e.g. a double-door entry or basic laboratory—Biosafety Level 2), describing a specific area designed to maintain the pressure differential between the laboratory and its adjacent space. The anteroom should have facilities for separating clean and dirty clothing and a shower may also be necessary.
2.  Anteroom doors may be self-closing and interlocking so that only one door is open at a time. A breakthrough panel may be provided for emergency exit use.
3.  Surfaces of walls, floors and ceilings should be water-resistant and easy to clean. Openings through these surfaces (e.g. for service pipes) should be sealed to facilitate decontamination of the room(s).
4.  The laboratory room must be sealable for decontamination. Air-ducting systems must be constructed to permit gaseous decontamination.
5.  Windows must be closed, sealed and break-resistant.
6.  A handwashing station with hands-free controls should be provided near each exit door.
7.  There must be a controlled ventilation system that maintains a directional airflow into the laboratory room. A visual monitoring device with or without alarm(s) should be installed so that staff can at all times ensure that proper directional airflow into the laboratory room is maintained.
8.  The building ventilation system must be so constructed that air from the containment laboratory, Biosafety Level 3 is not recirculated to other areas within the building. Air may be high-efficiency particulate air (HEPA) filtered, reconditioned and recirculated within that laboratory. When

exhaust air from the laboratory (other than from biological safety cabinets) is discharged to the outside of the building, it must be dispersed away from occupied buildings and air intakes. Depending on the agents in use, this air may be discharged through HEPA-filters. A heating, ventilation and air-conditioning (HVAC) control system may be installed to prevent sustained positive pressurization of the laboratory. Consideration should be given to the installation of audible or clearly visible alarms to notify personnel of HVAC system failure.

9. All HEPA-filters must be installed in a manner that permits gaseous decontamination and testing.

10. Biological safety cabinets should be sited away from walking areas and out of cross-currents from doors and ventilation systems.

11. The exhaust air from Class I or Class II biological safety cabinets, which will have been passed through HEPA-filters, must be discharged in such a way as to avoid interference with the air balance of the cabinet or the building exhaust system.

12. An autoclave for the decontamination of contaminated waste material should be available in the containment laboratory. If infectious waste has to be removed from the containment laboratory for decontamination and disposal, it must be transported in sealed, unbreakable and leak-proof containers according to national or international regulations, as appropriate.

13. Backflow-precaution devices must be fitted to the water supply. Vacuum lines should be protected with liquid disinfectant traps and HEPA-filters, or their equivalent. Alternative vacuum pumps should also be properly protected with traps and filters.

14. The containment laboratory, Biosafety Level 3 facility design and operational procedures should be documented.

## Laboratory Equipment

The principles for the selection of laboratory equipment, including biological safety cabinets are the same as for the basic laboratory—Biosafety Level 2. However, at Biosafety Level 3, manipulation of all potentially infectious material must be conducted within a biological safety cabinet or other primary containment device. Consideration should b e given to equipment such as centrifuges, which will need additional containment accessories, for example, safety buckets or containment rotors. Some centrifuges and other equipment, such as cell-sorting instruments for use with infected cells, may need additional local exhaust ventilation with HEPA filtration for efficient containment.

## Biosafety Level 4 (The Maximum Containment Laboratory)

The maximum containment laboratory, Biosafety Level 4 is designed for work with Risk Group 4 microorganisms. Before such a laboratory is constructed and put into operation, intensive consultations should be held with institutions that have had experience of operating a similar facility. Operational maximum containment laboratories, Biosafety Level 4 should be under the control of national or other appropriate health authorities. The following information is intended only as introductory material.

## Code of Practice

The code of practice for Biosafety Level 3 applies except where modified as follows:

1. The two-person rule should apply, whereby no individual ever works alone. This is particularly important if working in a Biosafety Level 4 suit facility.
2. A complete change of clothing and shoes is required prior to entering and upon exiting the laboratory.
3. Personnel must be trained in emergency extraction procedures in the event of personnel injury or illness.
4. A method of communication for routine and emergency contacts must be established between personnel working within the maximum containment laboratory, Biosafety Level 4 and support personnel outside the laboratory.

## Laboratory Design and Facilities

The features of a containment laboratory, Biosafety Level 3 also apply to a maximum containment laboratory, Biosafety Level 4 with the addition of the following:

1. **Primary containment**: An efficient primary containment system must be in place, consisting of one or a combination of the following:
   - *Class III cabinet laboratory:* Passage through a minimum of two doors prior to entering the rooms containing the Class III biological safety cabinet(s) (cabinet room) is required. In this laboratory configuration the Class III biological safety cabinet provides the primary containment. A personnel shower with inner and outer changing rooms is necessary. Supplies and materials that are not brought into the cabinet room through the changing area are introduced through a double-door autoclave or fumigation chamber. Once the outer door is securely closed, staff inside the laboratory can open the inner door to retrieve the materials. The doors of the autoclave or fumigation chamber are interlocked in such a way that the outer door cannot open unless the autoclave has been operated through a sterilization cycle or the fumigation chamber has been decontaminated.
   - *Suit laboratory:* A protective suit laboratory with self-contained breathing apparatus differs significantly in design and facility requirements from a Biosafety Level 4 laboratory with Class III biological safety cabinets. The rooms in the protective suit laboratory are arranged so as to direct personnel through the changing and decontamination areas prior to entering areas where infectious materials are manipulated.
   - A suit decontamination shower must be provided and used by personnel leaving the containment laboratory area. A separate personnel shower with inner and outer changing rooms is also provided. Personnel who enter the suit area are required to don a one-piece, positively pressurized, HEPA-filtered, supplied-air suit. Air to the suit must be provided by a system that has a 100% redundant capability with an independent source of air, for use in the event of an emergency. Entry into the suit laboratory is through an airlock fitted with airtight doors. An appropriate warning system for personnel working in the suit laboratory must be provided for use in the event of mechanical system or air failure.

2. **Controlled access**: The maximum containment laboratory, Biosafety Level 4 must be located in a separate building or in a clearly delineated zone within a secure building. Entry and exit of personnel and supplies must be through an airlock or pass-through system. On entering, personnel must put on a complete change of clothing; before leaving, they should shower before putting on their street clothing.

3. **Controlled air system**: Negative pressure must be maintained in the facility. Both supply and exhaust air must be HEPA-filtered. There are significant differences in the ventilating systems of the Class III cabinet laboratory and suit laboratory:

   - Class III cabinet laboratory: The supply air to the Class III biological safety cabinet(s) may be drawn from within the room through a HEPA-filter mounted on the cabinet or supplied directly through the supply air system. Exhaust air from the Class III biological safety cabinet must pass through two HEPA-filters prior to release outdoors. The cabinet must be operated at negative pressure to the surrounding laborator y at all times. A dedicated non-recirculating ventilating system for the cabinet laboratory is required.

   - Suit laboratory: Dedicated room air supply and exhaust systems are required.

     The supply and exhaust components of the ventilating system are balanced to provide directional airflow within the suit area from the area of least hazard to the area(s) of greatest potential hazard. Redundant exhaust fans are required to ensure that the facility remains under negative pressure at all times. The differential pressures within the suit laboratory and between the suit laboratory and adjacent areas must be monitored. Airflow in the supply and exhaust components of the ventilating system must be monitored, and an appropriate system of controls must be used to prevent pressurization of the suit laboratory. HEPA-filtered supply air must be provided to the suit area, decontamination shower and decontamination airlocks or chambers. Exhaust air from the suit laboratory must be passed through a series of two HEPA-filters prior to release outdoors. Alternatively, after double HEPA filtration, exhaust air may be recirculated, but only within the suit laboratory. Under no circumstances shall the exhaust air from the Biosafety Level 4 suit laboratory be recirculated to other areas. Extreme caution must be exercised if recirculation of air within the suit laboratory is elected. Consideration must be given to the types of research conducted, equipment, chemicals and other materials used in the suit laboratory, as well as animal species that may be involved in the research.

All HEPA-filters need to be tested and certified annually. The HEPA-filter housings are designed to allow for in situ decontamination of the filter prior to removal. Alternatively, the filter can be removed in a sealed, gas-tight primary container for subsequent decontamination and/or destruction by incineration.

4. **Decontamination of effluents**: All effluents from the suit area, decontamination chamber, decontamination shower, or Class III biological safety cabinet must be decontaminated before final discharge. Heat treatment is the preferred method. Effluents may also require correction

to a neutral pH prior to discharge. Water from the personnel shower and toilet may be discharged directly to the sanitary sewer without treatment.

5. **Sterilization of waste and materials:** A double-door, pass-through autoclave must be available in the laboratory area. Other methods of decontamination must be available for equipment and items that cannot withstand steam sterilization.

6. **Airlock entry ports:** For specimens, materials and animals must be provided.

7. **Emergency power** and dedicated power supply line(s) must be provided.

8. **Containment drain(s)** must be installed.

## PERSONAL PROTECTIVE EQUIPMENT AND CLOTHING

Personal protective equipment and clothing may act as a barrier to minimize the risk of exposure to aerosols, splashes and accidental inoculation. The clothing and equipment selected is dependent on the nature of the work performed. Protective clothing should be worn when working in the laboratory. Before leaving the laboratory, protective clothing should be removed, and hands should be washed.

### Laboratory Coats, Gowns, Coveralls, Aprons

Laboratory coats should preferably be fully-buttoned. However, long-sleeved, back- opening gowns or coveralls give better protection than laboratory coats and are preferred in microbiology laboratories and when working at the biological safety cabinet. Aprons may be worn over laboratory coats or gowns where necessary to give further protection against spillage of chemicals or biological materials such as blood or culture fluids. Laundering services should be provided at/near the facility. Laboratory coats, gowns, coveralls, or aprons should not be worn outside the laboratory areas (Table 1.2).

### Goggles, Safety Spectacles, Face Shields

The choice of equipment to protect the eyes and face from splashes and impacting objects will depend on the activity performed. Prescription or plain eye glasses can be manufactured with special frames that allow lenses to be placed in frame from the front, using shatterproof material either curved or fitted with side shields (safety glasses). Safety spectacles do not provide for adequate splash protection even when side shields are worn with them. Goggles for splash and impact protection should be worn over normal prescription eye glasses and contact lenses (which do not provide protection against biological or chemical hazards). Faces shields (visors) are made of shatterproof plastic fit over the face and are held in place by head straps or caps. Goggles, safety spectacles, or face shields should not be worn outside the laboratory areas.

### Respirators

Respiratory protection may be used when carrying out high hazard procedures (e.g. cleaning up a spill of infectious material). The choice of respirator will depend on the type of hazard(s). Respirators are available with interchangeable filters for protection against gases, vapors, particulates and microorganisms.

■ **Table 1.2** Personal protective equipment

| Equipment | Hazard corrected | Safety features |
|---|---|---|
| Laboratory coats, gowns, coveralls | Contamination of clothing | • Back opening<br>• Cover street clothing |
| Plastic aprons | Contamination of clothing | • Waterproof |
| Footwear | Impact and splash | • Closed-toe |
| Goggles | Impact and splash | • Impact-resistant lenses (must be optically correct or worn over corrective eye glasses) |
| | | • Side shields |
| Safety spectacles Impact | | • Impact-resistant lenses (must be optically correct) |
| | | • Side shields |
| Face shields | Impact and splash | • Shield entire face |
| | | • Easily removable in case of accident |
| Respirators | Inhalation of aerosols | • Designs available include single-use disposable; full-face or half-face air purifying; full-face or hooded powered air purifying (PAPR); and supplied air respirators |
| Gloves | Direct contact with microorganisms | • Disposable microbiologically approved latex, microorganisms vinyl or nitrile |
| | | • Hand protection |
| | Cuts | • Mesh |

## PROCEDURE OF PUTTING ON PERSONAL PROTECTIVE EQUIPMENT

### Laboratory coats, gowns, coveralls

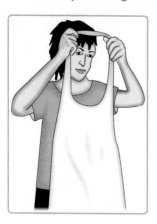

## Respiratory protection

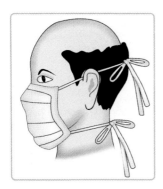 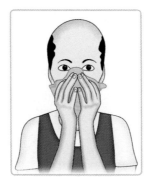

## Goggles or face shield

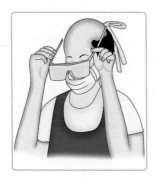 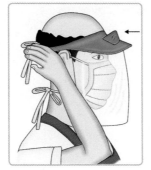

## Disposable gloves

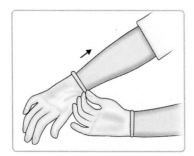

## PROCEDURE OF REMOVAL OF PERSONAL PROTECTIVE EQUIPMENT

### Gloves

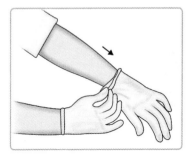 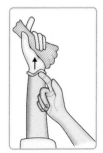

### Laboratory coats, gowns, coveralls

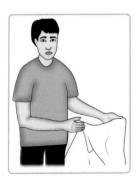

### Goggles or face shield

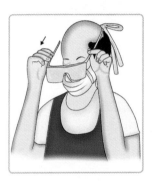

## Respiratory protection

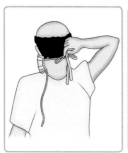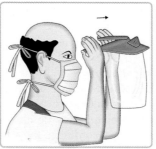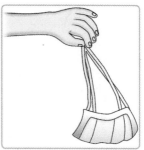

# LABORATORY ANIMAL FACILITIES

Those who use animals for experimental and diagnostic purposes have a moral obligation to take every care to avoid causing them unnecessary pain or suffering. The animals must be provided with comfortable, hygienic housing and adequate wholesome food and water. At the end of the experiment they must be dealt with in a humane manner.

For security reasons, the animal house should be an independent, detached unit. If it adjoins a laboratory, the design should provide for its isolation from the public parts of the laboratory should such need arise, and for its decontamination and disinfestation.

Animal facilities, like laboratories, may be designated according to a risk assessment and the risk group of the microorganisms under investigation, as Animal Facility Biosafety Level 1, 2, 3 or 4 (Table 1.3).

With respect to agents to be used in the animal laboratory, factors for consideration include:

1. The normal route of transmission.
2. The volumes and concentrations to be used.

**Table 1.3** Animal facility containment levels: summary of practices and safety equipment

| Risk group | Containment level | Laboratory practices and safety equipment |
|---|---|---|
| 1 | ABSL-1 | Limited access, protective clothing and gloves |
| 2 | ABSL-2 | ABSL-1 practices plus: Hazard warning signs. Class I or II BSCs for activities that produce aerosols Decontamination of waste and cages before washing |
| 3 | ABSL-3 | ABSL-2 practices plus: Controlled access. BSCs and special protective clothing for all activities |
| 4 | ABSL-4 | ABSL-3 plus: Strictly limited access. Clothing change before entering. Class III BSCs or positive pressure suits. Shower on exit. Decontamination of all wastes before removal from facility |

ABSL, Animal Facility Biosafety Level; BSCs, Biological Safety Cabinets

3. The route of inoculation.
4. Whether and by what route these agents may be excreted.

With respect to animals to be used in the animal laboratory, factors for consideration include:

1. The nature of the animals, i.e. their aggressiveness and tendency to bite and scratch.
2. Their natural ecto- and endoparasites.
3. The zoonotic diseases to which they are susceptible.
4. The possible dissemination of allergens.

As with laboratories, the requirements for design features, equipment and precautions increase in stringency according to the animal Biosafety Level.

These guidelines are additive, so that each higher level incorporates the standards of the lower levels.

## Animal Facility—Biosafety Level 1

This is suitable for the maintenance of most stock animals after quarantine (except nonhuman primates , regarding which national authorities should be consulted), and for animals that are deliberately inoculated with agents in Risk Group 1. GMT is required. The animal facility director must establish policies, procedures and protocols for all operations, and for access to the vivarium. An appropriate medical surveillance program for the staff must be instituted. A safety or operations manual must be prepared and adopted.

## Animal Facility—Biosafety Level 2

This is suitable for work with animals that are deliberately inoculated with micro-organisms in Risk Group 2. The following safety precautions apply:

1. All the requirements for animal facilities—Biosafety Level 1 must be met.
2. Biohazard warning signs should be posted on doors and other appropriate places.
3. The facility must be designed for easy cleaning and housekeeping.
4. Doors must open inwards and be self-closing.
5. Heating, ventilation and lighting must be adequate.
6. If mechanical ventilation is provided, the airflow must be inwards. Exhaust air is discharged to the outside and should not be recirculated to any part of the building.
7. Access must be restricted to authorized persons.
8. No animals should be admitted other than those for experimental use.
9. There should be an arthropod and rodent control program.
10. Windows, if present, must be secure, resistant to breakage and, if able to be opened, must be fitted with arthropod-proof screens.
11. After use, work surfaces must be decontaminated with effective disinfectants.
12. Biological safety cabinets (Classes I or II) or isolator cages with dedicated air supplies and HEPA-filtered exhaust air must be provided for work that may involve the generation of aerosols.
13. An autoclave must be available on site or in appropriate proximity to the animal facility.

14. Animal bedding materials must be removed in a manner that minimizes the generation of aerosols and dust.
15. All waste materials and bedding must be decontaminated before disposal.
16. Use of sharp instruments should be restricted whenever possible. Sharps should always be collected in puncture-proof/ resistant containers fitted with covers and treated as infectious.
17. Material for autoclaving or incineration must be transported safely, in closed containers.
18. Animal cages must be decontaminated after use.
19. Animal carcasses should be incinerated.
20. Protective clothing and equipment must be worn in the facility, and removed on leaving.
21. Hand-washing facilities must be provided. Staff must wash their hands before leaving the animal facility.
22. All injuries, however minor, must be treated appropriately, reported and recorded.
23. Eating, drinking, smoking and application of cosmetics must be forbidden in the facility.
24. All personnel must receive appropriate training.

## Animal Facility—Biosafety Level 3

This is suitable for work with animals that are deliberately inoculated with agents in Risk Group 3, or when otherwise indicated by a risk-assessment. All systems, practices and procedures need to be reviewed and recertified annually. The following safety precautions apply:

1. All the requirements for animal facilities—Biosafety Levels 1 and 2 must be met.
2. Access must be strictly controlled.
3. The facility must be separated from other laboratory and animal house areas by a room with a double-door entrance forming an anteroom.
4. Hand-washing facilities must be provided in the anteroom.
5. Showers should be provided in the anteroom.
6. There must be mechanical ventilation to ensure a continuous airflow through all the rooms. Exhaust air must pass through HEPA-filters before being discharged to the atmosphere without recirculation. The system must be designed to prevent accidental reverse flow and positive pressurization in any part of the animal house.
7. An autoclave must be available at a location convenient for the animal house where the biohazard is contained. Infectious waste should be autoclaved before it is moved to other areas of the facility.
8. An incinerator should be readily available on site or alternative arrangements should be made with the authorities concerned.
9. Animals infected with Risk Group 3 microorganisms must be housed in cages in isolators or rooms with ventilation exhausts placed behind the cages.
10. Bedding should be as dust-free as possible.
11. All protective clothing must be decontaminated before it is laundered.
12. Windows must be closed and sealed, and resistant to breakage.
13. Immunization of staff, as appropriate, should be offered.

### Animal Facility—Biosafety Level 4

Work in this facility will normally be linked with that in the maximum containment laboratory—Biosafety Level 4, and national and local rules and regulations must be harmonized to apply to both. If work is to be done in a suit laboratory, additional practices and procedures must be used over and above those described here:

1. All the requirements for animal facilities—Biosafety Levels 1, 2 and 3 must be met.
2. Access must be strictly controlled; only staff designated by the director of the establishment should have authority to enter.
3. Individuals must not work alone: the two-person rule must apply.
4. Personnel must have received the highest possible level of training as microbiologists and be familiar with the hazards involved in their work and with the necessary precautions.
5. Housing areas for animals infected with Risk Group 4 agents must maintain the criteria for containment described and applied for maximum containment laboratories—Biosafety Level 4.
6. The facility must be entered by an airlock anteroom, the clean side of which must be separated from the restricted side by changing and showering facilities.
7. Staff must remove street clothing when entering and put on special, protective clothing. After work they must remove the protective clothing for autoclaving, and shower before leaving.
8. The facility must be ventilated by a HEPA-filtered exhaust system designed to ensure a negative pressure (inward directional airflow).
9. The ventilation system must be designed to prevent reverse flow and positive-pressurization.
10. A double-ended autoclave with the clean end in a room outside the containment rooms must be provided for exchange of materials.
11. A pass-through airlock with the clean end in a room outside the containment rooms must be provided for exchange of non-autoclavable materials.
12. All manipulations with animals infected with Risk Group 4 agents must take place under maximum containment—Biosafety Level 4 conditions.
13. All animals must be housed in isolators.
14. All animal bedding and waste must be autoclaved before removal from the facility.
15. There must be medical supervision of staff.

### Invertebrates

As with vertebrates, the animal facility biosafety level will be determined by the risk groups of the agents under investigation or when otherwise indicated by a risk-assessment. The following additional precautions are necessary with certain arthropods, particularly with flying insects:

1. Separate rooms should be provided for infected and non-infected invertebrates.
2. The rooms should be capable of being sealed for fumigation.
3. Insecticide sprays should be readily available.
4. "Chilling" facilities should be provided to reduce, where necessary, the activity of invertebrates.

5.  Access should be through an anteroom containing insect traps and with arthropod-proof screens on the doors.
6.  All exhaust ventilation ducts and openable windows should be fitted with arthropod-proof screens.
7.  Waste traps on sinks and sluices should not be allowed to dry out.
8.  All waste should be decontaminated by autoclaving, as some invertebrates are not killed by all disinfectants.
9.  A check should be kept on the numbers of larval and adult forms of flying, crawling and jumping arthropods.
10. Containers for ticks and mites should stand in trays of oil.
11. Infected or potentially infected flying insects must be contained in double-netted cages.
12. Infected or potentially infected arthropods must be handled in biological safety cabinets or isolators.
13. Infected or potentially infected arthropods may be manipulated on cooling trays.

## LABORATORY EQUIPMENT

### Biological Safety Cabinets

Biological safety cabinets (BSCs) are designed to protect the operator, the laboratory environment and work materials from exposure to infectious aerosols and splashes that may be generated when manipulating materials containing infectious agents, such as primary cultures, stocks and diagnostic specimens. Aerosol particles are created by any activity that imparts energy into a liquid or semiliquid material, such as shaking, pouring, stirring or dropping liquid onto a surface or into another liquid. Other laboratory activities, such as streaking agar plates, inoculating cell culture flasks with a pipette, using a multi-channel pipette to dispense liquid suspensions of infectious agents into microculture plates, homogenizing and vortexing infectious materials, and centrifugation of infectious liquids, or working with animals, can generate infectious aerosols. Aerosol particles of less than 5 m in diameter and small droplets of 5–100 m in diameter are not visible to the naked eye. The laboratory worker is generally not aware that such particles are being generated and may be inhaled or may cross-contaminate work surface materials. BSCs, when properly used, have been shown to be highly effective in reducing laboratory-acquired infections and cross-contaminations of cultures due to aerosol exposures. BSCs also protect the environment.

Over the years the basic design of BSCs has undergone several modifications. A major change was the addition of a high-efficiency particulate air (HEPA) filter to the exhaust system. The HEPA-filter traps 99.97% of particles of 0.3 in diameter and 99.99% of particles of greater or smaller size. This enables the HEPA-filter to effectively trap all known infectious agents and ensure that only microbe-free exhaust air is discharged from the cabinet. A second design modification was to direct HEPA-filtered air over the work surface, providing protection of work surface materials from contamination. This feature is often referred to as product protection. These basic design concepts have led to the evolution of three classes of BSCs.

**Note:** Horizontal and vertical outflow cabinets ("clean-air work stations") are not biological safety cabinets and should not be used as such.

### Class I Biological Safety Cabinet

The directional flow of air whisks aerosol particles that may be generated on the work surface away from the laboratory worker and into the exhaust duct. The front opening allows the operator's arms to reach the work surface inside the cabinet while he or she observes the work surface through a glass window. The window can also be fully raised to provide access to the work surface for cleaning or other purposes (Table 1.4).

The air from the cabinet is exhausted through a HEPA-filter: (a) Into the laboratory and then to the outside of the building through the building exhaust; (b) To the outside through the building exhaust; or (c) Directly to the outside. The HEPA-filter may be located in the exhaust plenum of the BSC or in the building exhaust. Some Class I BSCs are equipped with an integral exhaust fan, whereas others rely on the exhaust fan in the building exhaust system.

The Class I BSC is the first recognized BSC and, because of its simple design, is still in wide use throughout the world. It has the advantage of providing personnel and environmental protection and can also be used for work with radionuclides and volatile toxic chemicals. Because unsterilized room air is drawn over the work surface through the front opening, it is not considered to provide consistently reliable product protection.

### Class II Biological Safety Cabinets

As the use of cell and tissue cultures for the propagation of viruses and other purposes grew, it was no longer considered satisfactory for unsterilized room air to pass over the work surface. The Class II BSC is designed not only to provide personnel protection but also to protect work surface materials from contaminated room air. Class II BSCs, of which there are four types (A1, A2,

**Table 1.4** Selection of a biological safety cabinet (BSC), by type of protection needed

| Type of protection | BSC selection |
|---|---|
| Personnel protection, microorganisms in Risk Groups 1–3 | Class I, Class II, Class III |
| Personnel protection, microorganisms in Risk Group 4, glove-box laboratory | Class III |
| Personnel protection, microorganisms in Risk Group 4, suit laboratory | Class I, Class II |
| Product protection | Class II, Class III only if laminar flow included |
| Volatile radionuclide/chemical protection, vented to the outside minute amounts | Class IIB1, Class IIA2 |
| Volatile radionuclide/chemical protection | Class I, Class IIB2, Class III |

B1 and B2), differ from Class I BSCs by allowing only air from a HEPA-filtered (sterile) supply to flow over the work surface. The Class II BSC can be used for working with infectious agents in Risk Groups 2 and 3. Class II BSCs can be used for working with infectious agents in Risk Group 4 when positive-pressure suits are used.

## Class II Type A1 Biological Safety Cabinet

The Class II type A1 BSC is internal fan draws room air (Supply air) into the cabinet through the front opening and into the front intake grill. The inflow velocity of this air should be at least 0.38 m/s at the face of the front opening. The supply air then passes through a supply HEPA-filter before flowing downwards over the work surface. As the air flows downwards it "splits" about 6–18 cm from the work surface, one half of the downwards flowing air passing through the front exhaust grill, and the other half passing through the rear exhaust grill. Any aerosol particles generated at the work surface are immediately captured in this downward airflow and passed through the front or rear exhaust grills, thereby providing the highest level of product protection. The air is then discharged through the rear plenum into the space between the supply and exhaust filters located at the top of the cabinet. Owing to the relative size of these filters, about 70% of the air recirculates through the supply HEPA-filter back into the work zone; the remaining 30% passes through the exhaust filter into the room or to the outside. Air from the Class IIA1 BSC exhaust can be recirculated to the room or discharged to the outside of the building through a thimble connection to a dedicated duct or through the building exhaust system (Figure 1.2).

Recirculating the exhaust air to the room has the advantage of lowering building fuel costs because heated and/or cooled air is not being passed to the outside environment. A connection to a ducted exhaust system also allows some BSCs to be used for work with volatile radionuclides and volatile toxic chemicals.

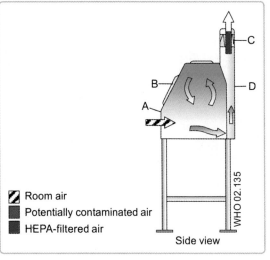

**Figure 1.2** Schematic diagram of a Class I biological safety cabinet. A. Front opening; B. Sash; C. Exhaust HEPA-filter; D. Exhaust plenum

C

B — D

A

WHO 02.135

- Room air
- Potentially contaminated air
- HEPA-filtered air

Side view

## Class II Type A2 Vented to the Outside, B1 and B2 Biological Safety Cabinets

Class IIA2 vented to the outside, IIB1 and IIB2 BSCs (Figure 1.4) are variations of the type IIA1. Their characteristics, along with those of Class I and Class III BSCs, are indicated (Figure 1.3). Each variation allows the BSC to be used for specialized purpose.

These BSCs differ from one another in several aspects: the air intake velocity through the front opening; the amount of air recirculated over the work surface and exhausted from the cabinet; the exhaust system, which determines whether air from the cabinet is exhausted to the room, or to the outside, through a dedicated exhaust system or through the building exhaust; and the pressure arrangements (whether cabinets have biologically contaminated ducts and plenums under negative pressure, or have biological contaminated ducts and plenums surrounded by negative-pressure ducts and plenums) (Table 1.5).

### Class III Biological Safety Cabinet

This type provides the highest level of personnel protection and is used for Risk Group 4 agents. All penetrations are sealed "gas tight". Supply air is HEPA-filtered and exhaust air passes through two HEPA-filters. Airflow is maintained by a dedicated exhaust system exterior to the cabinet, which keeps the cabinet interior under negative pressure (about 124.5 Pa). Access to the work surface is by means of heavy duty rubber gloves, which are attached to ports in the cabinet. The Class III BSC should have an attached pass-through box that can be sterilized and is equipped with a HEPA-filtered exhaust. The Class III cabinet may be connected to a double-door autoclave used to decontaminate all materials entering or exiting the cabinet. Several glove boxes can be joined together to extend the work surface. Class III BSCs are suitable for work in Biosafety Level 3 and 4 laboratories.

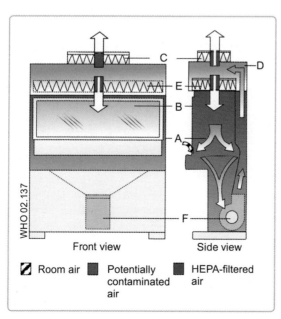

Front view    Side view

WHO 02.137

Room air    Potentially contaminated air    HEPA-filtered air

**Figure 1.3** Schematic representation of a Class IIA1 biological safety cabinet. A. Front opening; B. Sash; C. Exhaust HEPA-filter; D. Rear plenum; E. Supply HEPA-filter; F. Blower

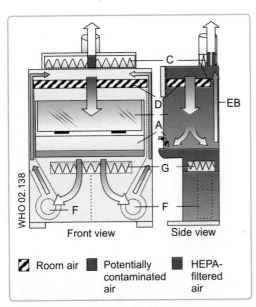

**Figure 1.4** Schematic diagram of a Class II B1 biological safety cabinet. A. Front opening; B. Sash; C. Exhaust HEPA-filter; D. Supply HEPA-filter; E. Negative-pressure exhaust plenum; F. Blower; G. HEPA-filter for supply air. Connection of the cabinet exhaust to the building exhaust air system is required

WHO 02.138

Front view    Side view

▨ Room air  ■ Potentially contaminated air  ■ HEPA-filtered air

■ **Table 1.5** Differences between Class I, II and III biological safety cabinets (BSCs)

| BSC | Face velocity (M/s) | Airflow (%) | | Exhaust system |
|---|---|---|---|---|
| | | Recirculated | Exhausted | |
| Class I[a] | 0.36 | 0 | 100 | Hard duct |
| Class IIA 1 | 0.38–0.51 | 70 | 30 | Exhaust to room or thimble connection |
| Class IIA 2 vented to the outside[a] | 0.51 | 70 | 30 | Exhaust to room or thimble connection |
| Class IIB 1[a] | 0.51 | 30 | 70 | Hard duct |
| Class IIB 2[a] | 0.51 | 0 | 100 | Hard duct |
| Class III[a] | NA | 0 | 100 | Hard duct |

NA, not applicable
[a] All biologically contaminated ducts are under negative pressure or are surrounded by negative pressure ducts and plenums

## Biological Safety Cabinet Air Connections

A "thimble" or "canopy hood" is designed for use with Class IIA1 and IIA2 vented to the outside BSCs. The thimble fits over the cabinet exhaust housing, sucking the cabinet exhaust air into the building exhaust ducts. A small opening, usually 2.5 cm in diameter, is maintained between the thimble and the cabinet exhaust housing. This small opening enables room air to be sucked into the building exhaust system as well.

The building exhaust capacity must be sufficient to capture both room air and the cabinet exhaust. The thimble must be removable or be designed to allow for operational testing of the cabinet. Generally, the performance of a thimble-connected BSC is not affected much by fluctuations in the airflow of the building Class IIB1 and IIB2 BSCs are hard-ducted, i.e. firmly connected without any openings, to the building exhaust system or, preferably, to a dedicated exhaust duct system. The building exhaust system must be precisely matched to the airflow requirements specified by the manufacturer for both volume and static pressure. Certification of hard-duct connected BSCs is more time-consuming than that for BSCs that recirculate air to the room or which are thimble-connected.

## Selection of a Biological Safety Cabinet

A BSC should be selected primarily in accordance with the type of protection needed: product protection, personnel protection against Risk Group 1–4 microorganisms, personnel protection against exposure to radionuclides and volatile toxic chemicals, or a combination of these. Table 8 shows which BSCs are recommended for each type of protection. Volatile or toxic chemicals should not be used in BSCs that recirculate exhaust air to the room, i.e. Class I BSCs that are not ducted to building exhaust systems, or Class IIA1 or Class IIA2 cabinets. Class IIB1 BSCs are acceptable for work with minute amounts of volatile chemicals and radionuclides. A Class IIB2 BSC, also called a total exhaust cabinet, is necessary when significant amounts of radionuclides and volatile chemicals are expected to be used (Figure 1.5).

## Using Biological Safety Cabinets in the Laboratory

### *Location*

The velocity of air flowing through the front opening into a BSC is about 0.45 m/s. At this velocity the integrity of the directional air inflow is fragile and

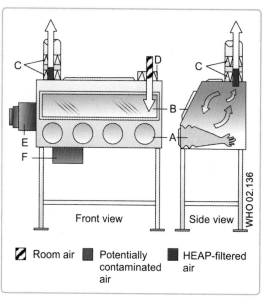

**Figure 1.5** Schematic representation of a Class III biological safety cabinet (glove box). A. Glove ports for arm-length gloves; B. Sash; C. Double-exhaust HEPA-filters; D. Supply HEPA-filter; E. Double-ended autoclave or pass-through box; F. Chemical dunk tank. Connection of the cabinet exhaust to an independent building exhaust airsystem is required

Front view    Side view

WHO 02.136

▨ Room air    ■ Potentially contaminated air    ■ HEAP-filtered air can be easily disrupted by air currents generated by people walking close to the BSC, open windows, air supply registers, and opening and shutting doors. Ideally, BSCs should be situated in a location remote from traffic and potentially disturbing air currents.

Whenever possible a 30 cm clearance should be provided behind and on each side of the cabinet to allow easy access for maintenance. A clearance of 30–35 cm above the cabinet may be required to provide for accurate air velocity measurement across the exhaust filter and for exhaust filter changes.

## Material Placement

The front intake grill of Class II BSCs must not be blocked with paper, equipment or other items. Materials to be placed inside the cabinet should be surface decontaminated with 70% alcohol. Work may be performed on disinfectant-soaked absorbent towels to capture splatters and splashes. All materials should be placed as far back in the cabinet, towards the rear edge of the work surface, as practical without blocking the rear grill. Aerosol-generating equipment (e.g. mixers, centrifuges, etc.) should be placed towards the rear of the cabinet. Bulky items, such as biohazard bags, discard pipette trays and suction collection flasks should be placed to one side of the interior of the cabinet. Active work should flow from clean to contaminated areas across the work surface.

The autoclavable biohazard collection bag and pipette collection tray should not be placed outside the cabinet. The frequent in-and-out movement needed to use these containers is disruptive to the integrity of the cabinet's air barrier, and can compromise both personnel and product protection.

## Ultraviolet Lights

Ultraviolet lights are not required in BSCs. If they are used, they must be cleaned weekly to remove any dust and dirt that may block the germicidal effectiveness of the light. Ultraviolet light intensity should be checked when the cabinet is recertified to ensure that light emission is appropriate. Ultraviolet lights must be turned off while the room is occupied, to protect eyes and skin from inadvertent exposure.

## Spills

A copy of the laboratory's protocol for handling spills should be posted, read and understood by everyone who uses the laboratory. When a spill of biohazardous material occurs within a BSC, clean-up should begin immediately, while the cabinet continues to operate. An effective disinfectant should be used and applied in a manner that minimizes the generation of aerosols. All materials that come into contact with the spilled agent should be disinfected and/or autoclaved.

## Cleaning and Disinfection

All items within BSCs, including equipment, should be surface-decontaminated and removed from the cabinet when work is completed, since residual culture media may provide an opportunity for microbial growth.

The interior surfaces of BSCs should be decontaminated before and after each use. The work surfaces and interior walls should be wiped with a disinfectant that will kill any microorganisms that might be found inside the cabinet. At the end of the work day, the final surface decontamination should include a wipe-down of the work surface, the sides, back and interior of the glass. A solution of bleach or 70% alcohol should be used where effective for target organisms. A second wiping with sterile water is needed when a corrosive disinfectant, such as bleach, is used.

It is recommended that the cabinet is left running. If not, it should be run for 5 minutes in order to purge the atmosphere inside before it is switched off.

### Decontamination

BSCs must be decontaminated before filter changes and before being moved. The most common decontamination method is by fumigation with formaldehyde gas. BSC decontamination should be performed by a qualified professional.

### Negative-Pressure Flexible-Film Isolators

The negative-pressure flexible-film isolator is a self-contained primary containment device that provides maximum protection against hazardous biological materials. It may be mounted on a mobile stand. The workspace is totally enclosed in a transparent polyvinylchloride (PVC) envelope suspended from a steel framework. The isolator is maintained at an internal pressure lower than atmospheric pressure. Inlet air is passed through one HEPA-filter and outlet air is passed through two HEPA-filters, thus obviating the need to duct exhaust air outside the building. The isolator may be fitted with an incubator, microscope and other laboratory equipment, such as centrifuges, animal cages, heat blocks, etc. Material is introduced and removed from the isolator through supply and sample ports without compromising microbiological security. Manipulations are performed using gloved sleeves incorporating disposable gloves. A manometer is installed to monitor envelope pressure.

Flexible-film isolators are used to manipulate high-risk organisms (Risk Groups 3 or 4) in field work where it is not feasible or appropriate to install or maintain conventional biological safety cabinets.

### Pipetting Aids

A pipetting aid must always be used for pipetting procedures. Mouth pipetting must be strictly forbidden. The importance of pipetting aids cannot be overemphasized. The most common hazards associated with pipetting procedures are the result of mouth suction. Oral aspiration and ingestion of hazardous materials have been responsible for many laboratory-associated infections.

Pathogens can also be transferred to the mouth if a contaminated finger is placed on the suction end of a pipette. A lesser known hazard of mouth pipetting is the inhalation of aerosols caused by suction. The cotton plug is not an efficient microbial filter at negative or positive pressure, and particles may be sucked through it. Violent suction may be applied when the plug is tightly packed, resulting in the aspiration of plug, aerosol and even liquid.

The ingestion of pathogens is prevented by the use of pipetting aids. Aerosols can also be generated when a liquid is dropped from a pipette on to a work surface, when cultures are mixed by alternate sucking and blowing, and when the last drop is blown out of a pipette. The inhalation of aerosols unavoidably generated during pipetting operations can be prevented by working in a biological safety cabinet. Pipetting aids should be selected with care. Their design and use should not create an additional infectious hazard and they should be easy to sterilize and clean. Plugged (aerosol-resistant) pipette tips should be used when manipulating microorganisms and cell cultures. Pipettes with cracked or chipped suction ends should not be used as they damage the seating seals of pipetting aids and so create a hazard.

## LABORATORY BIOSECURITY

Today the nation is facing a new challenge in safeguarding the public health from potential domestic or international terrorism involving the use of dangerous biological agents or toxins. Existing standards and practices may require adaptation to ensure protection from such hostile actions.

A specific laboratory biosecurity refers to institutional and personal security measures designed to protect workers, environment and population against the loss, theft, use and release in the environment of pathogenic biological agents and toxins. Biosecurity management and practices are designed to prevent the spread of disease by minimizing the movement of biologic organisms approaches enable staff to deal with the unpredicted and unfamiliar in the most prudent and safe manner.

A specific laboratory biosecurity protocol must be prepared and implemented for each facility according to the requirements of the facility, the type of laboratory work conducted, and the local conditions. Consequently, laboratory biosecurity activities should be representative of the institution's various needs and should include input from scientific directors, principal investigators, biosafety officers, laboratory scientific staff, maintenance staff, administrators, information technology staff, and law enforcement agencies and security staff if appropriate.

Laboratory biosecurity measures should be based on a comprehensive program of accountability for pathogens and toxins that includes an updated inventory with storage location, identification of personnel with access, description of use, documentation of internal and external transfers within and between facilities, and any inactivation and/or disposal of the materials. Likewise, an institutional laboratory biosecurity protocol should be established for identifying, reporting, investigating and remediating breaches in laboratory biosecurity, including discrepancies in inventory results. The involvement and roles and responsibilities of public health and security authorities in the event of a security infraction must be clearly defined.

Laboratory biosecurity training, distinct from laboratory biosafety training, should be provided to all personnel. Such training should help personnel understand the need for protection of such materials and the rationale for the specific biosecurity measures, and should include a review of relevant national standards and institution specific procedures.

Procedures describing the security roles and responsibilities of personnel in the event of a security infraction should also be presented during training. The professional and ethical suitability for working with dangerous pathogens of all personnel who have regular authorized access to sensitive materials is also central to effective laboratory biosecurity activities.

In summary, security precautions should become a routine part of laboratory work, just as have aseptic techniques and other safe microbiological practices. Laboratory biosecurity measures should not hinder the efficient sharing of reference materials, clinical and epidemiological specimens and related information necessary for clinical or public health investigations. Competent security management should not unduly interfere with the day-to-day activities of scientific personnel or be an impediment to conducting research. Legitimate access to important research and clinical materials must be preserved. Assessment of the suitability of personnel, security-specific training and rigorous adherence to pathogen protection procedures are reasonable means of enhancing laboratory biosecurity. All such efforts must be established and maintained through regular risk and threat assessments, and regular review and updating of procedures.

## LABORATORY TECHNIQUES

Human error, poor laboratory techniques and misuse of equipment cause the majority of laboratory injuries and work-related infections. This section provides a compendium of technical methods that are designed to avoid or minimize the most commonly reported problems of this nature.

### Safe Handling of Specimens in the Laboratory

Improper collection, transport and handling of specimens in the laboratory carry a risk of infection to the personnel involved.

### Specimen Containers

Specimen containers may be of glass or preferably plastic. They should be robust and should not leak when the cap or stopper is correctly applied. No material should remain on the outside of the container. Containers should be correctly labeled to facilitate identification. Specimen request or specification forms should not be wrapped around the containers but placed in separate, preferably waterproof envelopes.

### Transport of Specimens within the Facility

To avoid accidental leakage or spillage, secondary containers, such as boxes, should be used, fitted with racks so that the specimen containers remain upright. The secondary containers may be of metal or plastic, should be autoclavable or resistant to the action of chemical disinfectants, and the seal should preferably have a gasket. They should be regularly decontaminated.

### Receipt of Specimens

Laboratories that receive large numbers of specimens should designate a particular room or area for this purpose.

### Opening Packages

Personnel who receive and unpack specimens should be aware of the potential health hazards involved, and should be trained to adopt standard precautions, particularly when dealing with broken or leaking containers. Primary specimen containers should be opened in a biological safety cabinet. Disinfectants should be available.

## Use of Pipettes and Pipetting Aids

1.  A pipetting aid must always be used. Pipetting by mouth must be prohibited.
2.  All pipettes should have cotton plugs to reduce contamination of pipetting devices.
3.  Air should never be blown through liquid containing infectious agents.
4.  Infectious materials should not be mixed by alternate suction and expulsion through a pipette.
5.  Liquids should not be forcibly expelled from pipettes.
6.  Mark-to-mark pipettes are preferable to other types as they do not require expulsion of the last drop.
7.  Contaminated pipettes should be completely submerged in a suitable disinfectant contained in an unbreakable container. They should be left in the disinfectant for the appropriate length of time before disposal.
8.  A discard container for pipettes should be placed within the biological safety cabinet, not outside it.
9.  Syringes fitted with hypodermic needles must not be used for pipetting.
10. Devices for opening septum-capped bottles that allow pipettes to be used and avoid the use of hypodermic needles and syringes should be used.
11. To avoid dispersion of infectious material dropped from a pipette, an absorbent material should be placed on the working surface; this should be disposed of as infectious waste after use.

## Avoiding the Dispersal of Infectious Materials

1.  In order to avoid the premature shedding of their loads, microbiological transfer loops should have a diameter of 2–3 mm and be completely closed. The shanks should be not more than 6 cm in length to minimize vibration.
2.  The risk of spatter of infectious material in an open Bunsen burner flame should be avoided by using an enclosed electric micro-incinerator to sterilize transfer loops. Disposable transfer loops, which do not need to be re-sterilized, are preferable.
3.  Care should be taken when drying sputum samples, to avoid creating aerosols.
4.  Discarded specimens and cultures for autoclaving and/or disposal should be placed in leak proof containers, e.g. laboratory discard bags. Tops should be secured (e.g. with autoclave tape) prior to disposal into waste containers.
5.  Working areas must be decontaminated with a suitable disinfectant at the end of each work period.

## Use of Biological Safety Cabinets

1.  The use and limitations of biological safety cabinets should be explained to all potential users, with reference to national standards and relevant literature. Written protocols or safety or operations manuals should be issued to staff. In particular, it must be made clear that the cabinet will not protect the operator from spillage, breakage or poor technique.

2. The cabinet must not be used unless it is working properly.
3. The glass viewing panel must not be opened when the cabinet is in use.
4. Apparatus and materials in the cabinet must be kept to a minimum. Air circulation at the rear plenum must not be blocked.
5. Bunsen burners must not be used in the cabinet. The heat produced will distort the airflow and may damage the filters. An electric micro-incinerator is permissible but sterile disposable transfer loops are better.
6. All work must be carried out in the middle or rear part of the working surface and be visible through the viewing panel.
7. Traffic behind the operator should be minimized.
8. The operator should not disturb the airflow by repeated removal and reintroduction of his or her arms.
9. Air grills must not be blocked with notes, pipettes or other materials, as this will disrupt the airflow causing potential contamination of the material and exposure of the operator.
10. The surface of the biological safety cabinet should be wiped using an appropriate disinfectant after work is completed and at the end of the day.
11. The cabinet fan should be run for at least 5 minutes before beginning work and after completion of work in the cabinet.
12. Paperwork should never be placed inside biological safety cabinets.

## Avoiding Ingestion of Infectious Materials and Contact with Skin and Eyes

1. Disposable gloves should be worn. Laboratory workers should avoid touching their mouth, eyes and face.
2. Food and drink must not be consumed or stored in the laboratory.
3. No articles should be placed in the mouth; pens, pencils, chewing gum in the laboratory.
4. Cosmetics should not be applied in the laboratory.
5. The face, eyes and mouth should be shielded or otherwise protected during any operation that may result in the splashing of potentially infectious materials.

## Avoiding Injection of Infectious Materials

1. Accidental inoculation resulting from injury with broken or chipped glassware can be avoided through careful practices and procedures. Glassware should be replaced with plasticware whenever possible.
2. Accidental injection may result from sharps injuries e.g. with hypodermic needles (needle-sticks), glass Pasteur pipettes, or broken glass.
3. Needle-stick injuries can be reduced by: (a) Minimizing the use of syringes and needles (e.g. simple devices are available for opening septum stoppered bottles so that pipettes can be used instead of syringes and needles; or (b) Using engineered sharp safety devices when syringes and needles are necessary.
4. Needles should never be recapped. Disposable articles should be discarded into puncture-proof/resistant containers fitted with covers.
5. Plastic Pasteur pipettes should replace those made of glass.

## Separation of Serum

1. Only properly trained staff should be employed for this work.
2. Gloves and eye and mucous membrane protection should be worn.
3. Splashes and aerosols can only be avoided or minimized by good laboratory technique. Blood and serum should be pipetted carefully, not poured. Pipetting by mouth must be forbidden.
4. After use, pipettes should be completely submerged in suitable disinfectant. They should remain in the disinfectant for the appropriate time before disposal or washing and sterilization for reuse.
5. Discarded specimen tubes containing blood clots, etc. (with caps replaced) should be placed in suitable leak proof containers for autoclaving and/or incineration.
6. Suitable disinfectants should be available for clean-up of splashes and spillages.

## Use of Centrifuges

1. Satisfactory mechanical performance is a prerequisite of microbiological safety in the use of laboratory centrifuges.
2. Centrifuges should be operated according to the manufacturer's instructions.
3. Centrifuges should be placed at such a level that workers can see into the bowl to place buckets correctly.
4. Centrifuge tubes and specimen containers for use in the centrifuge should be made of thick-walled glass or preferably of plastic and should be inspected for defects before use.
5. Tubes and specimen containers should always be securely capped.
6. The buckets must be loaded, equilibrated, sealed and opened in a biological safety cabinet.
7. Buckets should be paired by weight and, with tubes in place, correctly balanced.
8. The amount of space that should be left between the level of the fluid and the rim of the centrifuge tube should be given in manufacturer's instructions.
9. Distilled water or alcohol (propanol, 70%) should be used for balancing empty buckets. Saline or hypochlorite solutions should not be used as they corrode metals.
10. Sealable centrifuge buckets (safety cups) must be used for microorganisms in Risk Groups 3 and 4.
11. When using angle-head centrifuge rotors, care must be taken to ensure that the tube is not overloaded as it might leak.
12. The interior of the centrifuge bowl should be inspected daily for staining or soiling at the level of the rotor. If staining or soiling are evident then the centrifugation protocols should be re-evaluated.
13. Centrifuge rotors and buckets should be inspected daily for signs of corrosion and for hair-line cracks.
14. Buckets, rotors and centrifuge bowls should be decontaminated after each use.

15. After use, buckets should be stored in an inverted position to drain the balancing fluid.
16. Infectious airborne particles may be ejected when centrifuges are used. These particles travel at speeds too high to be retained by the cabinet airflow if the centrifuge is placed in a traditional open-fronted Class I or Class II biological safety cabinet. Enclosing centrifuges in Class III safety cabinets prevents emitted aerosols from dispersing widely.

However, good centrifuge technique and securely capped tubes offer adequate protection against infectious aerosols and dispersed particles.

## Use of Homogenizers, Shakers, Blenders and Sonicators

1. Domestic (kitchen) homogenizers should not be used in laboratories as they may leak or release aerosols. Laboratory blenders and stomachers are safer.
2. Caps and cups or bottles should be in good condition and free from flaws or distortion. Caps should be well-fitting and gaskets should be in good condition.
3. Pressure builds up in the vessel during the operation of homogenizers, shakers and sonicators. Aerosols containing infectious materials may escape from between the cap and the vessel. Plastic, in particular, polytetrafluoroethylene (PTFE) vessels are recommended because glass may break, releasing infectious material and possibly wounding the operator.
4. When in use, homogenizers, shakers and sonicators should be covered by a strong transparent plastic casing. This should be disinfected after use. Where possible, these machines should be operated, under their plastic covers, in a biological safety cabinet.
5. At the end of the operation the containers should be opened in a biological safety cabinet.
6. Hearing protection should be provided for people using sonicators.

## Use of Tissue Grinders

1. Glass grinders should be held in absorbent material in a gloved hand. Plastic (PTFE) grinders are safer.
2. Tissue grinders should be operated and opened in a biological safety cabinet.

## Care and Use of Refrigerators and Freezers

1. Refrigerators, deep-freezers and solid carbon dioxide (dry-ice) chests should be defrosted and cleaned periodically, and any ampoules, tubes, etc. that have broken during storage removed. Face protection and heavy duty rubber gloves should be worn during cleaning. After cleaning, the inner surfaces of the cabinet should be disinfected.
2. All containers stored in refrigerators, etc. should be clearly labeled with the scientific name of the contents, the date stored and the name of the individual who stored them. Unlabeled and obsolete materials should be autoclaved and discarded.
3. An inventory must be maintained of the freezer's contents.
4. Flammable solutions must not be stored in a refrigerator unless it is explosion-proof. Notices to this effect should be placed on refrigerator doors.

## Opening of Ampoules Containing Lyophilized Infectious Materials

Care should be taken when ampoules of freeze-dried materials are opened, as the contents may be under reduced pressure and the sudden inrush of air may disperse some of the materials into the atmosphere. Ampoules should always be opened in a biological safety cabinet.

## Ampoules Opening Procedure

1. First decontaminate the outer surface of the ampoule.
2. Make a file mark on the tube near to the middle of the cotton or cellulose plug, if present.
3. Hold the ampoule in alcohol-soaked cotton to protect hands before breaking it at a file scratch.
4. Remove the top gently and treat as contaminated material.
5. If the plug is still above the contents of the ampoule, remove it with sterile forceps.
6. Add liquid for resuspension slowly to the ampoule to avoid frothing.

## Storage of Ampoules Containing Infectious Materials

Ampoules containing infectious materials should never be immersed in liquid nitrogen because cracked or imperfectly sealed ampoules may break or explode on removal. If very low temperatures are required, ampoules should be stored only in the gaseous phase above the liquid nitrogen. Otherwise, infectious materials should be stored in mechanical deep-freeze cabinets or on dry ice. Laboratory workers should wear eye and hand protection when removing ampoules from cold storage. The outer surfaces of ampoules stored in these ways should be disinfected when the ampoules are removed from storage.

Standard precautions with blood, another body fluids, tissues and excreta: Standard precautions are designed to reduce the risk of transmission of microorganisms from both recognized and unrecognized sources of infection.

## Collection, Labeling and Transport of Specimens

1. Standard precautions should always be followed; gloves should be worn for all procedures.
2. Blood should be collected from patients and animals by trained staff.
3. For phlebotomies, conventional needle and syringe systems should be replaced by single-use safety vacuum devices that allow the collection of blood directly into stoppered transport and/or culture tubes, automatically disabling the needle after use.
4. The tubes should be placed in adequate containers for transport to the laboratory and within the laboratory facility (see section on Transport of specimens within the facility in this chapter). Request forms should be placed in separate waterproof bags or envelopes.
5. Reception staff should not open these bags.

## *Opening Specimen Tubes and Sampling Contents*

1. Specimen tubes should be opened in a biological safety cabinet.

2. Gloves must be worn. Eye and mucous membrane protection is also recommended (goggles or face shields).
3. Protective clothing should be supplemented with a plastic apron.
4. The stopper should be grasped through a piece of paper or gauze to prevent splashing.

## Films and Smears for Microscopy

Fixing and staining of blood, sputum and fecal samples for microscopy do not necessarily kill all organisms or viruses on the smears. These items should be handled with forceps, stored appropriately, and decontaminated and/or autoclaved before disposal.

## Automated Equipment (Sonicators, Vortex Mixers)

1. Equipment should be of the closed type to avoid dispersion of droplets and aerosols.
2. Effluents should be collected in closed vessels for further autoclaving and/ or disposal.
3. Equipment should be disinfected at the end of each session, following manufacturers' instructions.

## Tissues

1. Formalin fixatives should be used.
2. Frozen sectioning should be avoided. When necessary, the cryostat should be shielded and the operator should wear a safety face shield. For decontamination, the temperature of the instrument should be raised to at least 20°C.

## Decontamination

Hypochlorites and high-level disinfectants are recommended for decontamination. Freshly prepared hypochlorite solutions should contain available chlorine at 1 g/L for general use and 5 g/L for blood spillages. Glutaraldehyde may be used for decontaminating surfaces.

## Precautions with Materials that may Contain Prions

Prions (also referred to as "slow viruses") are associated with the transmissible spongiform encephalopathies (TSEs), notably Creutzfeldt-Jakob disease (CJD; including the new variant form), Gerstmann-Sträussler-Scheinker syndrome, fatal familial insomnia and kuru in humans; scrapie in sheep and goats; bovine spongiform encephalopathy (BSE) in cattle; and other transmissible encephalopathies of deer, elk and mink. Although CJD has been transmitted to humans, there appear to be no proven cases of laboratory-associated infections with any of these agents. Nevertheless, it is prudent to observe certain precautions in the handling of material from infected or potentially infected humans and animals.

The selection of a biosafety level for work with materials associated with TSEs will depend on the nature of the agent and the samples to be studied, and should be undertaken in consultation with national authorities.

The highest concentrations of prions are found in central nervous system tissue. Animal studies suggest that it is likely that high concentrations of prions are also found in the spleen, thymus, lymph nodes and lung. Recent studies indicate that prions in lingual and skeletal muscle tissue may also present a potential infection risk. As complete inactivation of prions is difficult to achieve, it is important to stress the use of disposable instruments whenever possible, and to use a disposable protective covering for the work surface of the biological safety cabinet.

The main precaution to be taken is to avoid ingestion of contaminated materials or puncture of the laboratory worker's skin. The following additional precautions should be taken, as the agents are not killed by the normal processes of laboratory disinfection and sterilization.

1.  The use of dedicated equipment, i.e. equipment not shared with other laboratories, is highly recommended.
2.  Disposable laboratory protective clothing (gowns and aprons) and gloves must be worn (steel mesh gloves between rubber gloves for pathologists).
3.  Use of disposable plastic ware, which can be treated and discarded as dry waste, is highly recommended.
4.  Tissue processors should not be used because of the problems of disinfection. Jars and beakers (plastic) should be used instead.
5.  All manipulations must be conducted in biological safety cabinets.
6.  Great care should be exercised to avoid aerosol production, ingestion, and cuts and punctures of the skin.
7.  Formalin-fixed tissues should be regarded as still infectious, even after prolonged exposure to formalin.
8.  Histological samples containing prions are substantially inactivated after exposure to 96% formic acid for 1 hour
9.  Bench waste, including disposable gloves, gowns and aprons, should be autoclaved using a porous load steam sterilizer at 134–137°C for a single cycle of 18 minutes or six successive cycles of 3 minutes each, followed by incineration.
10. Non-disposable instruments, including steel mesh gloves, must be collected for decontamination.
11. Infectious liquid waste contaminated with prions should be treated with sodium hypochlorite containing available chlorine at 20 g/L (2%) (final concentration) for 1 hour.
12. Paraformaldehyde vaporization procedures do not diminish prion titers and prions are resistant to ultraviolet irradiation. However, the cabinets must continue to be decontaminated by standard methods (i.e. formaldehyde gas) to inactivate other agents that may be present.
13. Prion-contaminated biological safety cabinets and other surfaces can be decontaminated with sodium hypochlorite containing available chlorine at 20 g/L (2%) for 1 hour.
14. High-efficiency particulate air (HEPA) filters should be incinerated at a Minimum temperature of 1000°C after removal.

Recommended additional steps prior to incineration include:
•   Spraying of the exposed face of the filter with lacquer hairspray prior to removal

- "Bagging" of filters during removal.
- Removal of the HEPA-filters from the working chamber so that the inaccessible plenum of the cabinet is not contaminated.
15. Instruments should be soaked in sodium hypochlorite containing available chlorine at 20 g/L (2%) for 1 hour and then rinsed well in water before autoclaving.
16. Instruments that cannot be autoclaved can be cleaned by repeated wetting with sodium hypochlorite containing available chlorine at 20 g/L (2%) over a 1-hour period. Appropriate washing to remove residual sodium hypochlorite is required.

## PACKING AND TRANSPORTATION OF INFECTIOUS SUBSTANCES

Transport of infectious and potentially infectious materials is subject to strict national and international regulations. These regulations describe the proper use of packaging materials, as well as other shipping requirements. Laboratory personnel must ship infectious substances according to applicable transport regulations. Compliance with the rules will:

1. Reduce the likelihood that packages will be damaged and leak, and thereby,
2. Reduce the exposures resulting in possible infections
3. Improve the efficiency of package delivery. The International Air Transport Association (IATA) issues *Infectious Substances Shipping Guidelines* every year. IATA guidelines must follow ICAO's *Technical Instructions* as a minimal standard, but may impose additional restrictions. IATA guidelines must be followed if a shipment is carried by members of IATA.

Since the United Nations *Model Regulations on the Transport of Dangerous Goods* is a dynamic set of recommendations subject to biennial amendments, the reader is referred to the latest issuances of national and international modal regulations for applicable regulatory texts.

### Infectious Substances

Defined as substances which are known or are reasonably expected to contain pathogens. Pathogens are defined as microorganisms (including bacteria, viruses, rickettsiae, parasites, fungi) and other agents such as prions which can cause disease in humans or animals (Table 1.6 and Figure 1.7).

- **Category A** (UN 2814 and UN 2900): An infectious substance which is transported in a form that, when exposure to it occurs, is capable of causing permanent disability, life-threatening or fatal disease in otherwise healthy humans or animals.
- **Category B** (UN 3373): An infectious substance that does not meet the criteria for Category A (Figure 1.8 for packaging such specimens).
- **Exemptions:** The following are exempt from these regulations:
  - Substances containing microorganisms which are non-pathogenic to humans or animals e.g. Hazard Group 1 agents.

■ **Table 1.6** Category A infectious substances

| UN number and Proper shipping name | Microorganism |
|---|---|
| UN 2814 infectious substances affecting humans | *Bacillus anthracis* (cultures only)<br>*Brucella abortus* (cultures only), *Brucella melitensis* (cultures only)<br>*Brucella suis* (cultures only), *Burkholderia mallei - Pseudomonas mallei*—Glanders (cultures only)<br>*Burkholderia pseudomalleii – Pseudomonas pseudomalleii* (cultures only)<br>*Chlamydia psittaci*—avian strains (cultures only)<br>*Clostridium botulinum* (cultures only)<br>*Coccidioides immitis* (cultures only)<br>*Coxiella burnetii* (cultures only)<br>Crimean-Congo hemorrhagic fever virus<br>Dengue virus (cultures only)<br>Eastern equine encephalitis virus (cultures only)<br>*Escherichia coli*, verotoxigenic (cultures only)<br>Ebola virus<br>Flexal virus<br>*Francisella tularensis* (cultures only)<br>Guanarito virus<br>Hantaan virus<br>Hantaviruses causing hemorrhagic fever with renal syndrome ‡<br>Hendra virus<br>Hepatitis B virus (cultures only)<br>Herpes B virus (cultures only)<br>Human immunodeficiency virus (cultures only)<br>Highly pathogenic avian influenza virus (cultures only)<br>Japanese encephalitis virus (cultures only)<br>Junin virus<br>Kyasanur forest disease virus<br>Lassa virus<br>Machupo virus<br>Marburg virus<br>Monkeypox virus<br>*Mycobacterium tuberculosis* (cultures only)<br>Nipah virus<br>Omsk hemorrhagic fever virus<br>Poliovirus (cultures only)<br>Rabies virus (cultures only) ‡<br>*Rickettsia prowazekii* (cultures only)<br>*Rickettsia rickettsii* (cultures only)<br>Rift Valley fever virus (cultures only) ‡<br>Russian spring-summer encephalitis virus (cultures only)<br>Sabia virus<br>*Shigella dysenteriae* type 1 (cultures only)<br>Tick-borne encephalitis virus (cultures only)<br>Variola virus<br>Venezuelan equine encephalitis virus<br>West Nile virus (cultures only)<br>Yellow fever virus (cultures only)<br>*Yersinia pestis* (cultures only) |

*Contd...*

*Contd...*

| UN 2900 infectious substances affecting animals only | African swine fever virus (cultures only)<br>Avian paramyxovirus Type 1 - Velogenic Newcastle disease virus (cultures only) ‡<br>Classical swine fever virus (cultures only) ‡<br>Foot and mouth disease virus (cultures only) ‡<br>Lumpy skin disease virus (cultures only) ‡<br>Mycoplasma mycoides - Contagious bovine pleuropneumonia (cultures only) ‡<br>Peste des petits ruminants virus (cultures only) ‡<br>Rinderpest virus (cultures only) ‡<br>Sheep-pox virus (cultures only) ‡<br>Goat-pox virus (cultures only) ‡<br>Swine vesicular disease virus (cultures only) ‡<br>Vesicular stomatitis virus (cultures only) ‡ |
|---|---|

- Substances transported in a form whereby any pathogens present have been neutralized or inactivated such that they no longer pose a health risk e.g. substances fixed in formaldehyde.
- Environmental samples (including food and water) which are not considered to pose a significant risk of infection.

## Marking and Labeling

The package must include the following:
- The proper shipping name, e.g. 'Infectious substance, affecting humans'
- Consignor and consignee addresses
- UN specification markings
- UN ID number and proper shipping name of contents
- The actual name of the infectious agent in brackets after the proper shipping name (no longer required for air transport), the name and telephone number (24 hours) of the person responsible for the shipment.
- The Class 6.2 (infectious substance) hazard warning diamond.
- The appropriate UN number (For example, 'Infectious substances, affecting humans' this would be UN 2814)
- The appropriate warning label (Figure 1.6).

## The Triple Packaging System

Transport of infectious substances requires a basic triple packaging system. It consists of three layers as follows:
- Primary receptacle: A primary watertight leak-proof receptacle containing the specimen. The receptacle is packaged with enough absorbent material to absorb all fluid in case of breakage (Figure 1.7).
- Secondary packaging: A second durable, watertight, leak-proof packaging to enclose and protect the primary receptacle(s) (Figure 1.8). Several cushioned primary receptacles may be placed in one secondary packaging, but sufficient additional absorbent material shall be used to absorb all fluid in case of breakage.

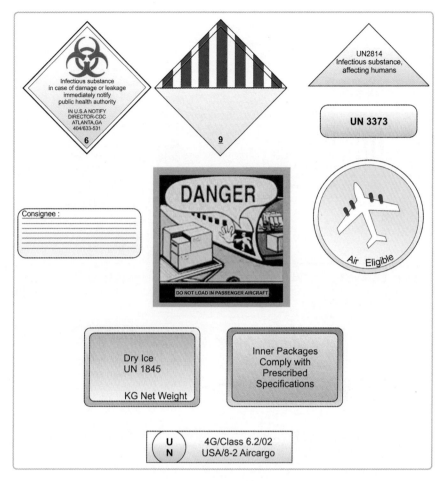

**Figure 1.6** Packaging warning signs

- Outer packaging: Secondary packaging is placed in outer shipping packaging with suitable cushioning material. Outer packaging protects contents from outside influences, such as physical damage, while in transit.

Each completed package is normally required to be marked, labeled and accompanied with appropriate shipping which is available from the Department for Transport.

## Spill Clean-up Procedure

In the event of a spill of infectious or potentially infectious material, the following spill clean-up procedure should be used.

1. Wear gloves and protective clothing, including face and eye protection if indicated.
2. Cover the spill with cloth or paper towels to contain it.
3. Pour an appropriate disinfectant over the paper towels and the immediately surrounding area (generally, 5% bleach solutions are appropriate; but for spills on aircraft, quaternary ammonium disinfectants should be used).

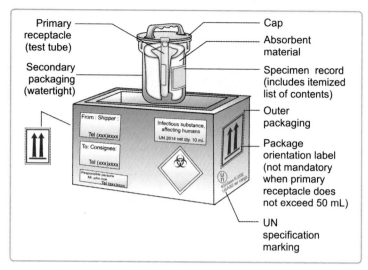

**Figure 1.7** Packing and labeling of category A infectious substances

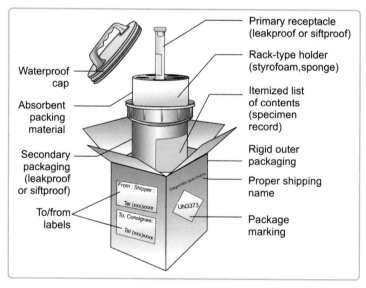

**Figure 1.8** Packing and labeling of category B infectious substances

4. Apply disinfectant concentrically beginning at the outer margin of the spill area, working toward the center.
5. After the appropriate amount of time (e.g. 30 minutes), clear away the materials. If there is broken glass or other sharps involved, use a dustpan or a piece of stiff cardboard to collect the material and deposit it into a puncture-resistant container for disposal.
6. Clean and disinfect the area of the spillage (if necessary, repeat steps 2–5).
7. Dispose of contaminated materials into a leak proof, puncture resistant waste disposal container.

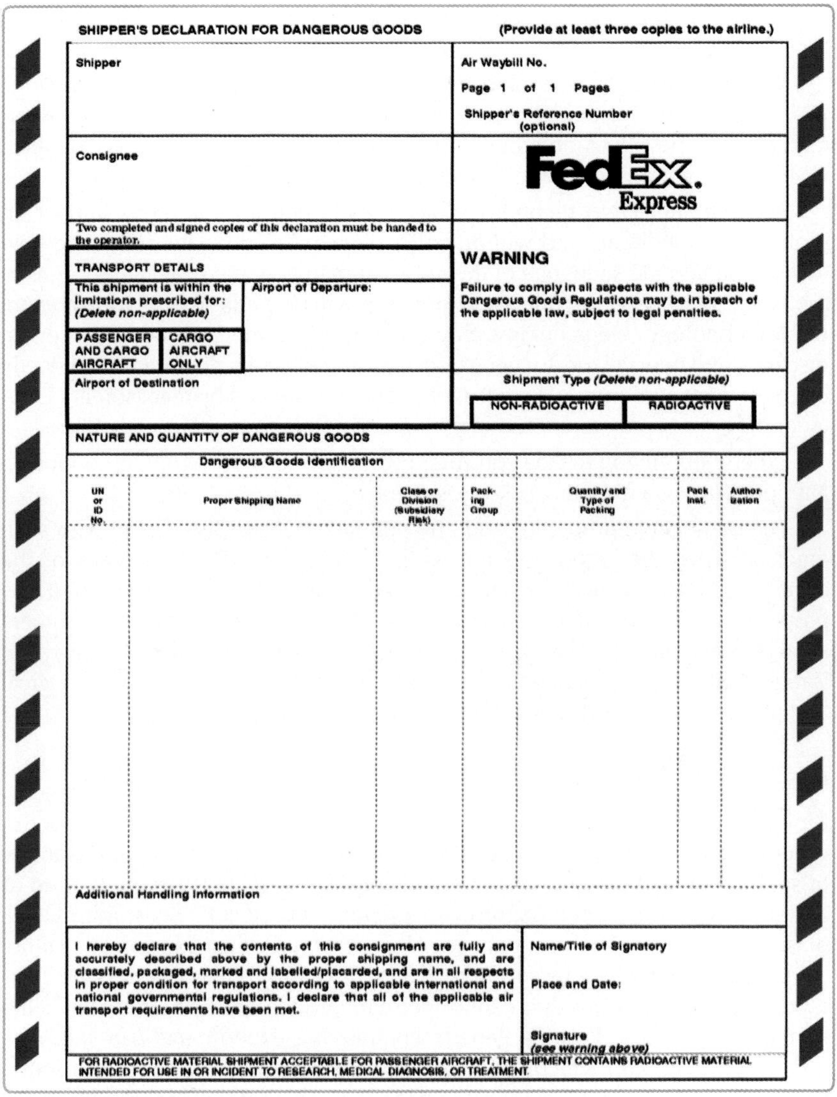
SHIPPER'S DECLARATION FOR DANGEROUS GOODS (Provide at least three copies to the airline.)

Shipper

Air Waybill No.

Page 1 of 1 Pages

Shipper's Reference Number (optional)

Consignee

FedEx. Express

Two completed and signed copies of this declaration must be handed to the operator.

TRANSPORT DETAILS

This shipment is within the limitations prescribed for: *(Delete non-applicable)*

PASSENGER AND CARGO AIRCRAFT | CARGO AIRCRAFT ONLY

Airport of Departure:

Airport of Destination

WARNING

Failure to comply in all aspects with the applicable Dangerous Goods Regulations may be in breach of the applicable law, subject to legal penalties.

Shipment Type *(Delete non-applicable)*

NON-RADIOACTIVE | RADIOACTIVE

NATURE AND QUANTITY OF DANGEROUS GOODS

| Dangerous Goods Identification | | | | | | |
|---|---|---|---|---|---|---|
| UN or ID No. | Proper Shipping Name | Class or Division (Subsidiary Risk) | Packing Group | Quantity and Type of Packing | Pack Inst. | Authorization |

Additional Handling Information

I hereby declare that the contents of this consignment are fully and accurately described above by the proper shipping name, and are classified, packaged, marked and labelled/placarded, and are in all respects in proper condition for transport according to applicable international and national governmental regulations. I declare that all of the applicable air transport requirements have been met.

Name/Title of Signatory

Place and Date:

Signature
*(see warning above)*

FOR RADIOACTIVE MATERIAL SHIPMENT ACCEPTABLE FOR PASSENGER AIRCRAFT, THE SHIPMENT CONTAINS RADIOACTIVE MATERIAL INTENDED FOR USE IN OR INCIDENT TO RESEARCH, MEDICAL DIAGNOSIS, OR TREATMENT.

**Figure 1.9** Shipper's declaration for dangerous goods example

8. After successful disinfection, inform the competent authority that the site has now been decontaminated.

**Figure 1.9 shows Shippers declaration format.**

## BIOSAFETY AND BIOTECHNOLOGY

Recombinant DNA technology involves combining genetic material from different sources thereby creating genetically modified organisms (GMOs) that may have never existed in nature before. Initially, there was concern among molecular biologists that such organisms might have unpredictable and undesirable properties that could represent a biohazard if they escaped from the laboratory.

Recombinant DNA technology or genetic engineering was first used to clone DNA segments in bacterial hosts in order to overexpress specific gene products for further studies. Recombinant DNA molecules have also been used to create GMOs such as transgenic and "knock-out" animals and transgenic plants.

Recombinant DNA technology has already had an enormous impact on biology and medicine, and will probably have an even greater influence now that the nucleotide sequence of the entire human genome is available. Tens of thousands of genes of yet unknown functions will be studied using recombinant DNA technology. Genetherapy may become a routine treatment for certain diseases, and new vectors for gene transfer are likely to be devised using genetic engineering techniques. Also, transgenic plants produced by recombinant DNA technology may play an increasingly important role in modern agriculture.

Experiments involving the construction or use of GMOs should be conducted after performing a biosafety risk-assessment.

The pathogenic properties and any potential hazards associated with such organisms may be novel and not well-characterized. The properties of the donor organism, the nature of the DNA sequences that will be transferred, the properties of the recipient organism, and the properties of the environment should be evaluated. These factors should help determine the biosafety level that is required for the safe handling of the resulting GMO, and identify the biological and physical containment systems that should be used.

## Biosafety Considerations for Biological Expression Systems

Biological expression systems consist of vectors and host cells. A number of criteria must be satisfied to make them effective and safe to use. An example of such a biological expression system is plasmid pUC18. Frequently used as a cloning vector in combination with *Escherichia coli* K12 cells, the pUC18 plasmid has been entirely sequenced. All genes required for expression in other bacteria have been deleted from its precursor plasmid pBR322. *E. coli* K12 is a non-pathogenic strain that cannot permanently colonize the gut of healthy humans or animals. Routine genetic engineering experiments can safely be performed in *E. coli* K12/pUC18 at Biosafety Level 1 provided the inserted foreign DNA expression products do not require higher biosafety levels.

## Biosafety Considerations for Expression Vectors

Higher biosafety levels may be required when:
1. The expression of DNA sequences derived from pathogenic organisms may increase the virulence of the GMO.
2. Inserted DNA sequences are not well-characterized, e.g. during preparation of genomic DNA libraries from pathogenic microorganisms.
3. Gene products have potential pharmacological activity.
4. Gene products code for toxins.

## Viral Vectors for Gene Transfer

Viral vectors, e.g. adenovirus vectors, are used for the transfer of genes to other cells. Such vectors lack certain virus replication genes and are propagated in cell lines that complement the defect. Stocks of such vectors may be contaminated with replication-competent viruses, generated by rare spontaneous recombination events in the propagating cell lines, or may derive from insufficient purification. These vectors should be handled at the same biosafety level as the parent adenovirus from which they are derived.

## Transgenic and "Knock-Out" Animals

Animals carrying foreign genetic material (transgenic animals) should be handled in containment levels appropriate to the characteristics of the products of the foreign genes. Animals with targeted deletions of specific genes ("knock-out"animals) do not generally present particular biological hazards.

Examples of transgenic animals include animals expressing receptors for viruses normally unable to infect that species. If such animals escaped from the laboratory and transmitted the transgene to the wild animal population, an animal reservoir for that particular virus could theoretically be generated.

This possibility has been discussed for poliovirus and is particularly relevant in the context of poliomyelitis eradication. Transgenic mice expressing the human poliovirus receptor generated in different laboratories were susceptible to poliovirus infection by various inoculation routes and the resulting disease was clinically and histopathologically similar to human poliomyelitis. However, the mouse model differs from humans in that alimentary tract replication of orally administered poliovirus is either inefficient or does not occur. It is, therefore, very unlikely that escape of such transgenic mice to the wild would result in the establishment of a new animal reservoir for poliovirus. Nevertheless, this example indicates that, for each new line of transgenic animal, detailed studies should be conducted to determine the routes by which the animals can be infected, the inoculum size required for infection, and the extent of virus shedding by the infected animals. In addition, all measures should be taken to assure strict containment of receptor transgenic mice.

## Transgenic Plants

Transgenic plants expressing genes that confer tolerance to herbicides or resistance to insects are currently a matter of considerable controversy in many parts of the world. The discussions focus on the food-safety of such plants, and on the long-term ecological consequences of their cultivation. Transgenic plants expressing genes of animal or human origin are used to develop medicinal and nutritional products. A risk-assessment should determine the appropriate biosafety level for the production of these plants.

## Risk-Assessments for Genetically Modified Organisms

Risk-assessments for work with GMOs should consider the characteristics of donor and recipient/host organisms. Examples of characteristics for consideration include the following:

### Hazards Arising Directly from the Inserted Gene (Donor Organism)

Assessment is necessary in situations where the product of the inserted gene has known biologically or pharmacologically active properties that may give rise to harm, for example:

1. Toxins
2. Cytokines
3. Hormones
4. Gene expression regulators
5. Virulence factors or enhancers
6. Oncogenic gene sequences
7. Antibiotic resistance
8. Allergens.

The consideration of such cases should include an estimation of the level of expression required to achieve biological or pharmacological activity.

## Hazards Associated with the Recipient/Host

1. Susceptibility of the host.
2. Pathogenicity of the host strain, including virulence, infectivity and toxin production.
3. Modification of the host range.
4. Recipient immune status.
5. Consequences of exposure.

## Hazards Arising from the Alteration of Existing Pathogenic Traits

Many modifications do not involve genes whose products are inherently harmful, but adverse effects may arise as the result of alteration of existing non-pathogenic or pathogenic traits. Modification of normal genes may alter pathogenicity. In an attempt to identify these potential hazards, the following points may be considered (the list is not exhaustive).

1. Is there an increase in infectivity or pathogenicity?
2. Could any disabling mutation within the recipient be overcome as a result of the insertion of the foreign gene?
3. Does the foreign gene encode a pathogenicity determinant from another organism?
4. If the foreign DNA does include a pathogenicity determinant, is it foreseeable that this gene could contribute to the pathogenicity of the GMO?
5. Is treatment available?
6. Will the susceptibility of the GMO to antibiotics or other forms of therapy be affected as a consequence of the genetic modification?
7. Is eradication of the GMO achievable?

### Further Considerations

The use of whole animals or plants for experimental purposes also requires careful consideration.

Investigators must comply with the regulations, restrictions and requirements for the conduct of work with GMOs in host countries and institutions. Countries may have national authorities that establish guidelines for work with GMOs, and may help scientists classify their work at the appropriate biosafety level. In some cases classification may differ between countries, or countries may decide to classify work at a lower or higher level when new information on a particular vector/ host system becomes available.

Risk-assessment is a dynamic process that takes into account new developments and the progress of science. The performance of appropriate risk-assessments will assure that the benefits of recombinant DNA technology remain available to human kind in the years to come.

# DISINFECTION AND STERILIZATION

A basic knowledge of disinfection and sterilization is crucial for biosafety in the laboratory. Since heavily soiled items cannot promptly be disinfected or sterilized, it is equally important to understand the fundamentals of cleaning prior to disinfection (precleaning). In this regard, the following general principles apply to all known classes of microbial pathogens.

Specific decontamination requirements will depend on the type of experimental work and the nature of the infectious agent(s) being handled. The generic information given here can be used to develop both standardized and more specific procedures to deal with biohazard(s) involved in a particular laboratory.

Contact times for disinfectants are specific for each material and manufacturer. Therefore, all recommendations for use of disinfectants should follow manufacturers' specifications.

## Definitions

Many different terms are used for disinfection and sterilization. The following are among the more common in biosafety:

### Antimicrobial

An agent that kills microorganisms or suppresses their growth and multiplication.

### Antiseptic

A substance that inhibits the growth and development of microorganisms without necessarily killing them. Antiseptics are usually applied to body surfaces.

### Biocide

A general term for any agent that kills organisms.

### Chemical Germicide

A chemical or a mixture of chemicals used to kill microorganisms.

### Decontamination

Any process for removing and/or killing microorganisms. The same term is also used for removing or neutralizing hazardous chemicals and radioactive materials.

### Disinfectant

A chemical or mixture of chemicals used to kill microorganisms, but not necessarily spores. Disinfectants are usually applied to inanimate surfaces or objects.

### Disinfection

A physical or chemical means of killing microorganisms, but not necessarily spores.

### Microbicide

A chemical or mixture of chemicals that kills microorganisms. The term is often used in place of "biocide", "chemical germicide" or "antimicrobial".

### Sporocide

A chemical or mixture of chemicals used to kill microorganisms and spores.

### Sterilization

A process that kills and/or removes all classes of microorganisms and spores.

## Cleaning Laboratory Materials

Cleaning is the removal of dirt, organic matter and stains. Cleaning includes brushing, vacuuming, drydusting, washing or damp mopping with water containing a soap or detergent. Dirt, soil and organic matter can shield microorganisms and can interfere with the killing action of decontaminants (antiseptics, chemical germicides and disinfectants). Precleaning is essential to achieve proper disinfection or sterilization.

Many germicidal products claim activity only on precleaned items. Precleaning must be carried out with care to avoid exposure to infectious agents.

Materials chemically compatible with the germicides to be applied later must be used. It is quite common to use the same chemical germicide for precleaning and disinfection.

## Local Environmental Decontamination

Decontamination of the laboratory space, its furniture and its equipment requires a combination of liquid and gaseous disinfectants. Surfaces can be decontaminated using a solution of sodium hypochlorite (NaOCl); a solution containing 1 g/L available chlorine may be suitable for general environmental sanitation, but stronger solutions (5 g/L) are recommended when dealing with high-risk situations. For environmental decontamination, formulated solutions containing 3% hydrogen peroxide ($H_2O_2$) make suitable substitutes for bleach solutions.

Rooms and equipment can be decontaminated by fumigation with formaldehyde gas generated by heating paraformaldehyde or boiling formalin.

This is a highly dangerous process that requires specially trained personnel. All openings in the room (i.e. windows, doors, etc.) should be sealed with masking tape or similar before the gas is generated. Fumigation should be conducted at an ambient temperature of at least 21°C and a relative humidity of 70%.

After fumigation the area must be ventilated thoroughly before personnel are allowed to enter. Appropriate respirators must be worn by anyone entering the room before it has been ventilated. Gaseous ammonium bicarbonate can be used to neutralize the formaldehyde. Fumigation of smaller spaces with hydrogen peroxide vapor is also effective but requires specialized equipment to generate the vapor.

## Decontamination of Biological Safety Cabinets

To decontaminate Class I and Class II cabinets, equipment that independently generates, circulates and neutralizes formaldehyde gas is available. Alternatively, the appropriate amount of paraformaldehyde (final concentration of 0.8% paraformaldehyde in air) should be placed in a frying pan on an electric hot plate. Another frying pan, containing 10% more ammonium bicarbonate than paraformaldehyde, on a second hot plate is also placed inside the cabinet. The hot plate leads are plugged in outside the cabinet, so that operation of the pans can be controlled from the outside by plugging and unplugging the hot plates as necessary. If the relative humidity is below 70%, an open container of hot water should also be placed inside the cabinet before the front closure is sealed in place with strong tape (e.g. duct tape).

Heavy gauge plastic sheeting is taped over the front opening and exhaust port to make sure that the gas cannot seep into the room. Penetration of the electric leads passing through the front closure must also be sealed with duct tape.

The plate for the paraformaldehyde pan is plugged in. It is unplugged when all the paraformaldehyde has vaporized. The cabinet is left undisturbed for at least 6 hours.

The plate for the second pan is then plugged in and the ammonium bicarbonate is allowed to vaporize. This plate is then unplugged and the cabinet blower is switched on for two intervals of approximately 2 seconds each to allow the ammonium bicarbonate gas to circulate. The cabinet should be left undisturbed for 30 minutes before the front closure (or plastic sheeting) and the exhaust port sheeting are removed. The cabinet surfaces should be wiped down to remove residues before use.

## Handwashing/Hand Decontamination

Whenever possible, suitable gloves should be worn when handling biohazardous materials. However, this does not replace the need for regular and proper hand-washing by laboratory personnel. Hands must be washed after handling bio-hazardous materials and animals, and before leaving the laboratory.

In most situations, thorough washing of hands with ordinary soap and water is sufficient to decontaminate them, but the use of germicidal soaps is recommended in high-risk situations. Hands should be thoroughly lathered with soap, using friction, for at least 10 seconds, rinsed in clean water and dried using a clean paper or towel. Foot or elbow-operated faucets are recommended. Where not fitted, a paper/cloth towel should be used to turn-off the faucet handles to avoid recontaminating washed hands. As mentioned above, alcohol-based hand-rubs may be used to decontaminate lightly soiled hands when proper hand-washing is not available.

## How to Perform Handwashing

1. Remove jewelry (rings, bracelets) and watches.
2. Rinse hands and wrists under water.

3. Apply soap.
4. Using friction, wash hands for at least 10–15 seconds cleaning between fingers, nail beds, palms, back of hands, wrists and forearms. If hands are visibly soiled, more time may be requires.
5. Routine hand washing may be performed with any soap. Plain soap with water can physically remove a certain level of microbes, reduce and maintain minimal counts of colonizing flora as well as to mechanically removing the contaminating flora.
6. If there is no assistant to close the tap, cover the tap with fresh tissue paper and gently close. Taking care to see that the hand does not come in contact with unsterile tap.
7. Handwashing technique charts are displayed near sinks and can be followed (Figure 1.10).

Additional alcohol-based solutions (HICC approved hand rub) are recommended for use in setting where handwashing facilities are inadequate or inaccessible and hands are not visibly soiled. If these solutions are used as a substitute for handwashing, handwashing with soap and water should be performed as soon as possible after procedure.

### Improper Handwashing

It is not always possible to protect the skin against various contaminants in the workplace. Therefore, cleaning and taking care of the hands is an important part of developing a proactive, holistic stance against work related skin disorders.

However, for any organization, implementing and maintaining appropriate hand hygiene practices is a daily challenge as there are inconsistent hand hygiene habits across the population:

• Separate washroom studies from around the world show that only 70% of people wash their hands and only 30% of people actually use soap when washing their hands.
• People do not wash their hands frequently or adequately enough.
• The average person washes their hands for around 10 seconds. This will remove around 90% of germs from their hands.
• Bacteria grow and double in number in less than 20 minutes (Figure 1.11).

### Heat Disinfection and Sterilization

Heat is the most common among the physical agents used for the decontamination of pathogens. "Dry" heat, which is totally non-corrosive, is used to process many items of laboratory ware which can withstand temperatures of 160° or higher for 2–4 hours. Burning or incineration (Figures 1.12 and 1.13) is also a form of dry heat. "Moist" heat is most effective when used in the form of autoclaving.

Boiling does not necessarily kill all microorganisms and/or pathogens, but it may be used as the minimum processing for disinfection where other methods (chemical disinfection or decontamination, autoclaving) are not applicable or available. Sterilized items must be handled and stored such that they remain uncontaminated until used.

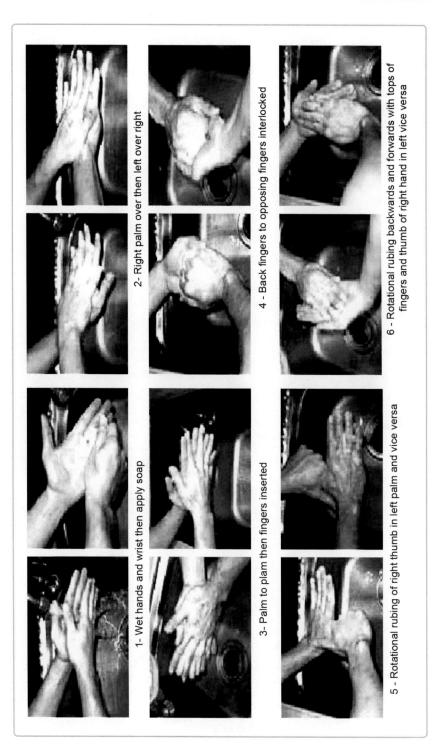

1- Wet hands and wrist then apply soap

2- Right palm over then left over right

3- Palm to plam then fingers inserted

4 - Back fingers to opposing fingers interlocked

5 - Rotational rubing of right thumb in left palm and vice versa

6 - Rotational rubing backwards and forwards with tops of fingers and thumb of right hand in left vice versa

**Figure 1.10** Handwash method

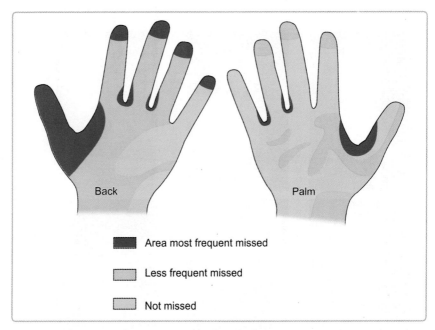

**Figure 1.11** Handwash—areas usually not washed properly

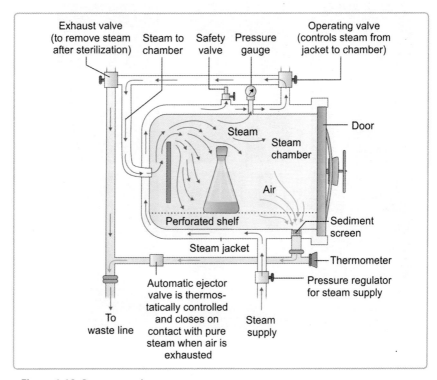

**Figure 1.12** Proper autoclave use

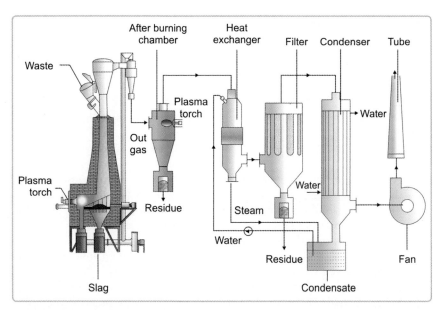

**Figure 1.13** Incinerator

## Autoclaving

Saturated steam under pressure (autoclaving) is the most effective and reliable means of sterilizing laboratory materials. For most purposes, the following cycles will ensure sterilization of correctly loaded autoclaves:

1. 3 minutes holding time at 134°C.
2. 10 minutes holding time at 126°C.
3. 15 minutes holding time at 121°C.
4. 25 minutes holding time at 115°C.

## Gravity Displacement Autoclave

- **Prevacuum autoclaves:** These machines allow the removal of air from the chamber before steam is admitted. The exhaust air is evacuated through a valve fitted with a HEPA-filter. At the end of the cycle, the steam is automatically exhausted.

    These autoclaves can operate at 134°C and the sterilization cycle can therefore be reduced to 3 minutes. They are ideal for porous loads, but cannot be used to process liquids because of the vacuum.

- **Fuel-heated pressure cooker autoclaves:** These should be used only if a gravity displacement autoclave is not available. They are loaded from the top and heated by gas, electricity or other types of fuels. Steam is generated by heating water in the base of the vessel, and air is displaced upwards through a relief vent. When all the air has been removed, the valve on the relief vent is closed and the heat reduced. The pressure and temperature rise until the safety valve operates at a preset level. This is the start of the holding time. At the end of the cycle the heat is turned-off and the temperature allowed to fall to 80°C or below before the lid is opened.

### Loading Autoclaves

Materials should be loosely packed in the chamber for easy steam penetration and air removal. Bags should allow the steam to reach their contents.

### Precautions in the Use of Autoclaves

The following rules can minimize the hazards inherent in operating pressurized vessels:

1. Responsibility for operation and routine care should be assigned to trained individuals.
2. A preventive maintenance program should include regular inspection of the chamber, door seals and all gauges and controls by qualified personnel.
3. The steam should be saturated and free from chemicals (e.g. corrosion inhibitors) that could contaminate the items being sterilized.
4. All materials to be autoclaved should be in containers that allow ready removal of air and permit good heat penetration; the chamber should be loosely packed so that steam will reach the load evenly.
5. For autoclaves without an interlocking safety device that prevents the door being opened when the chamber is pressurized, the main steam valve should be closed and the temperature allowed falling below 80°C before the door is opened.
6. Slow exhaust settings should be used when autoclaving liquids, as they may boil over when removed due to superheating.
7. Operators should wear suitable gloves and visors for protection when opening the autoclave, even when the temperature has fallen below 80°C.
8. In any routine monitoring of autoclave performance, biological indicators or thermocouples should be placed at the center of each load. Regular monitoring with thermocouples and recording devices in a "worst case" load is highly desirable to determine proper operating cycles.
9. The drain screen filter of the chamber (if available) should be removed and cleaned daily.
10. Care should be taken to ensure that the relief valves of pressure cooker autoclaves do not become blocked by paper, etc. in the load (Figure 1.12).

### Incineration

Incineration is useful for disposing of animal carcasses as well as anatomical and other laboratory waste, with or without prior decontamination. Incineration of infectious materials is an alternative to autoclaving only if the incinerator is under laboratory control.

Proper incineration requires an efficient means of temperature control and a secondary burning chamber. Many incinerators, especially those with a single combustion chamber, are unsatisfactory for dealing with infectious materials, animal carcasses and plastics. Such materials may not be completely destroyed and the effluent from the chimney may pollute the atmosphere with microorganisms, toxic chemicals and smoke. However, there are many satisfactory configuration s for combustion chambers. Ideally, the temperature in the primary chamber should be at least 800°C and that in the secondary chamber at least 1000°C. Materials for incineration, even with prior decontamination, should be transported to the incinerator in bags, preferably plastic. Incinerator attendants should receive proper instructions about loading and temperature control. It should also be noted that the efficient operation of an incinerator depends heavily on the right mix of materials in the waste being treated (Figure 1.13).

There are ongoing concerns regarding the possible negative environmental effects of existing or proposed incinerators, and efforts continue to make incinerators more environmentally friendly and energy efficient.

### Disposal

The disposal of laboratory and medical waste is subject to various regional, national and international regulations, and the latest versions of such relevant documents must be consulted before designing and implementing a program for handling, transportation and disposal of biohazardous waste. In general, ash from incinerators may be handled as normal domestic waste and removed by local authorities. Autoclaved waste may be disposed of by off-site incineration or in licensed land fill sites.

## THE BIOSAFETY OFFICER AND BIOSAFETY COMMITTEE

It is essential that each laboratory organization has a comprehensive safety policy, a safety manual, and supporting programs for their implementation. The responsibility for this normally rests with the director or head of the institute or laboratory, who may delegate certain duties to a biosafety officer or other appropriate personnel.

Laboratory safety is also the responsibility of all supervisors and laboratory employees, and individual workers are responsible for their own safety and that of their colleagues. Employees are expected to perform their work safely and should report any unsafe acts, conditions or incidents to their supervisor. Periodic safety audits by internal or external personnel are desirable.

### Biosafety Officer

Wherever possible a biosafety officer should be appointed to ensure that biosafety policies and programs are followed consistently throughout the laboratory. The biosafety officer executes these duties on behalf of the head of the institute or laboratory. In small units, the biosafety officer may be a microbiologist or a member of the technical staff, who may perform these duties on a defined part-time basis.

Whatever the degree of involvement in biosafety, the person designated should possess the professional competence necessary to suggest, review and approve specific activities that follow appropriate biocontainment and biosafety procedures. The biosafety officer should apply relevant national and international rules, regulations and guidelines, as well as assist the laboratory in developing standard operating procedures. The person appointed must have a technical background in microbiology, biochemistry and basic physical and biological sciences. Knowledge of laboratory and clinical practices and safety, including containment equipment, and engineering principles relevant to the design, operation and maintenance of facilities is highly desirable. The biosafety officer should also be able to communicate effectively with administrative, technical and support personnel.

The activities of the biosafety officer should include the following:

1.  Biosafety, biosecurity and technical compliance consultations.
2.  Periodic internal biosafety audits on technical methods, procedures and protocols, biological agents, materials and equipment.
3.  Discussions of violation of biosafety protocols or procedures with the appropriate persons.
4.  Verification that all staff has received appropriate biosafety training.
5.  Provision of continuing education in biosafety.
6.  Investigation of incidents involving the possible escape of potentially infectious or toxic material, and reporting of findings and recommendations to the laboratory director and biosafety.
7.  Coordination with medical staff regarding possible laboratory-acquired infections.
8.  Ensuring appropriate decontamination following spills or other incidents involving infectious material(s).
9.  Ensuring proper waste management.
10. Ensuring appropriate decontamination of any apparatus prior to repair or servicing.
11. Maintaining awareness of community attitudes regarding health and environmental considerations.
12. Establishment of appropriate procedures for import/export of pathogenic material to/from the laboratory, according to national regulations.
13. Reviewing the biosafety aspects of all plans, protocols and operating procedures for research work involving infectious agents prior to the implementation of these activities.
14. Institution of a system to deal with emergencies.

## Biosafety Committee

A biosafety committee should be constituted to develop institutional biosafety policies and codes of practice. The biosafety committee should also review research protocols for work involving infectious agents, animal use, recombinant DNA and genetically modified materials. Other functions of the committee may include risk assessments, formulation of new safety policies and arbitration in disputes over safety matters.

The membership of the biosafety committee should reflect the diverse occupational areas of the organization as well as its scientific expertise. The composition of a basic biosafety committee may include:

1.  Biosafety officer(s)
2.  Scientists
3.  Medical personnel
4.  Veterinarian(s) (if work with animals is conducted)
5.  Representatives of technical staff
6.  Representatives of laboratory management.

The biosafety committee should seek advice from different departmental and specialist safety officers (e.g. with expertise in radiation protection, industrial safety, fire prevention, etc.) and may at times require assistance from independent experts in various associated fields, local authorities and national regulatory bodies.

Community members may also be helpful if there is a particularly contentious or sensitive protocol under discussion.

## Immunization of Staff

The risks of working with particular agents should be fully discussed with individual researchers. The local availability, licensing state and utility of possible vaccines and/ or therapeutic drugs (e.g. antibiotic treatments) in case of exposure should be evaluated before work with such agents is started. Some workers may have acquired immunity from prior vaccination or infection.

If a particular vaccine or toxoid is locally licensed and available, it should be offered after a risk assessment of possible exposure and a clinical health assessment of the individual have been carried out.

Facilities for specific clinical case management following accidental infections should also be available.

## EMERGENCY SERVICES: WHOM TO CONTACT

The telephone numbers and addresses of the following should be prominently displayed in the facility:

- Director of the institution or laboratory
- Laboratory supervisor
- Biosafety officer
- Hospitals/ambulance
- Medical officer.

# Chapter Two

# Chemical Hazard

## INTRODUCTION

It is important that the laboratory staff have proper knowledge about 'Safety measures' about chemicals handling, proper storage, chemical spills and clean up, chemical burns, toxic effects, routes of exposure and the hazards that may be associated with chemicals to ensure that employees are protected from harm due to chemicals.

The terms "chemical accident" refer to an event resulting in the release of a substance or substances hazardous to human health and/or the environment in the short or long-term. Such events include fires, explosions, leakages or releases of toxic or hazardous materials that can cause people illness, injury, disability or death. Efforts should be applied to prevent accidents range by improving safety systems to fundamental changes in chemical use.

## CHEMICAL SAFETY LEVELS

- **Low risk (CSL-1):** Any chemical risk is usually managed by restricting usage of hazardous chemicals. Typically instrument laboratories and equipment laboratories do not use hazardous chemicals openly but rather in sealed vials or containers for use inside various analytical instruments.
- **Moderate risk (CSL-2):** Laboratories that use select carcinogens, reproductive toxins, or highly toxic chemicals. At this level, risk is still usually managed by restricting or limiting the quantities and volume of extremely hazardous chemicals allowed. This level includes laboratories that frequently use biological agents in association with various chemicals.
- **Substantial risk (CSL-3):** These laboratories typically work with a wide range of extremely hazardous chemicals or activities that may be, for example, very flammable, highly toxic, carcinogenic, teratogenic, or reactive. CSL-3 laboratories may use chemical hazard class 3 or 4 materials.
- **High risk (CSL-4):** The CSL-4 laboratory is a very special purpose laboratory that deals with hazardous chemicals where there is a high-risk of potential exposure to highly hazardous chemicals. These laboratories might involve production or isolation of high-hazard chemicals (Figure 2.1 and Table 2.1).

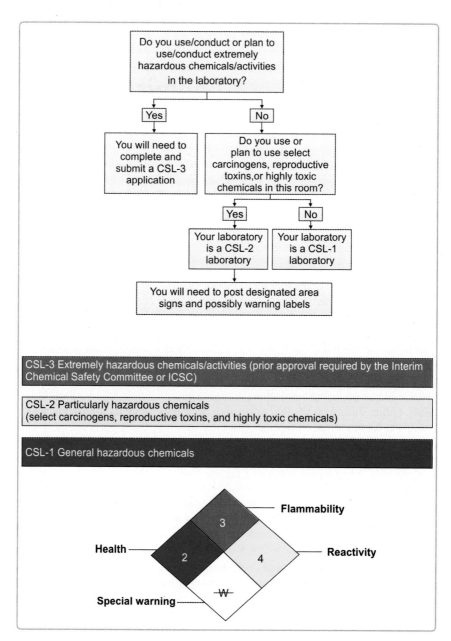

**Figure 2.1** Warning signs indication

**Post laboratory:** An appropriate sign must be posted on the outside of the main door to the laboratory. Emergency contact information must be posted on the inside of all doors to the laboratory and near the phone (see Emergency Contact Information Poster).

**Table 2.1** Health hazard color codes, flammability susceptibility and reactivity susceptibility of different materials

| Health Hazard Type of possible injury Color code: Blue | Flammability Susceptibility of Materials to burning Color code: Red | Reactivity Susceptibility to release energy Color code: Yellow |
|---|---|---|
| 4 Materials which on very short exposure could cause death or major residual injury even though prompt medical treatment was given | 4 Materials which will rapidly or completely vaporize at atmospheric pressure and normal ambient temperature, or which are readily dispersed in air and which will burn readily | 4 Materials which in themselves are readily capable of detonation or of explosive decomposition or reaction at normal temperatures and pressures |
| 3 Materials which on short exposure could cause serious temporary or residual injury even through prompt medical treatment was given | 3 Liquids and solids that can be ignited under almost all ambient temperature conditions | 3 Materials which in themselves are capable of detonation or of explosive reaction but require a strong initiating source or which must be heated under confinement before initiation or which react explosively with water |
| 2 Materials which on intense or continued exposure could cause serious temporary incapacitation or possible residual injury unless prompt medical treatment was given | 2 Materials that must be moderately heated or exposed to relatively high ambient temperatures before ignition can occur | 2 Materials which in themselves are normally unstable and readily undergo violent chemical change but do not detonate. Also materials which may react violently with water or which may form potentially explosive mixtures with water |
| 1 Materials which on exposure could cause serious temporary incapacitation or possible residual injury even if medical treatment is given | 1 Materials that must be preheated before ignition can occur | 1 Materials which in themselves are normally stable, but which can become unstable at elevated temperatures and pressures or which may react with water with some release of energy, but not violently |
| 0 Materials which on exposure under fire conditions would offer no hazard beyond that of ordinary combustible material | 0 Materials that will not burn | 0 Materials which in themselves are normally stable, even under fire exposure conditions, and which are not reactive with water |

## CHEMICAL SAFETY SYMBOLS

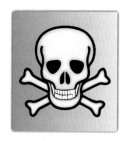

### Poisonous

Very hazardous to health when inhaled, swallowed or when they come in contact with the skin. May even lead to death. Danger! Avoid contact with the human body and immediately contact a physician in case of contact.

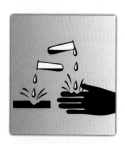

### Corrosive

Will destroy or irreversibly damage another substance with which it comes in contact. The main hazards include damage to eyes; skin and tissue under the skin, but inhalation or ingestion are also very risky. Avoid contact, and bear in mind that these can (under some circumstances) rust chemical cupboards.

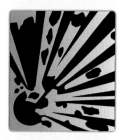

### Explosive

Self-explanatory, though fairly seldom seen in the average laboratory. Bear in mind that noise and movement can also trigger explosion (not just sparks/flames!).

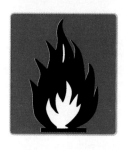

### Flammable or Extremely Flammable

Designates those items which are:
1. Flammable liquids—Caution! Flash point below 141°F (60.5°C).
2. Flammable solids—Caution! Keep away from open fires, sources of heat and sparks.
3. Combustible material—Caution! Flash point greater than 141°F but less than 200°F (or greater than 60.5°C but less than 90°C).

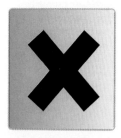

### Irritant or Harmful

This symbol covers a wide range of (sometimes relatively minor) hazards-with precautions such as avoid contact with the skin, do not breathe, etc. best to refer to relevant data sheet for details.

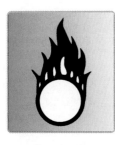

### Oxidizing Chemical

Oxidizing substances can ignite flammable and combustible material or worsen existing fire and thus make firefighting more difficult. Caution! Keep away from flammable, combustible and spontaneously combustible materials

Whereas the square symbols above (which tend to be the most familiar ones) will be found on bottles and jars, diamond shaped symbols are used in transport (mainly as they can be slotted into holders on the backs of trucks and tankers to identify what the mess is (and how dangerous it is) in the event of a leak.

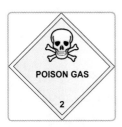

### Poisonous Gas

Used for transport of a poisonous gas—on gas cylinders, or sometimes as an indicator on vehicles.

### Miscellaneous Danger

Catch-all symbol for all other dangers (usually specified in the space).

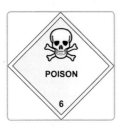

### Poison

More general symbol for the transport of poisonous materials (not necessarily a gas).

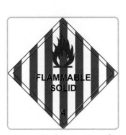

### Flammable Solid

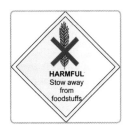

### Stow Away from Foodstuffs

Harmful material to be kept away from edible material.

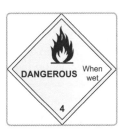

### Dangerous when Wet

This generally means that it will react fairly violently with water.

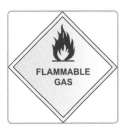

### Flammable Gas

Safety symbol used for the transport or storage of a flammable gas.

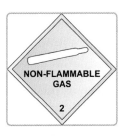

### Non-Flammable Gas

Safety symbol used in the transport of non-flammable (and hence often non-hazardous, at least out in the open) gases.

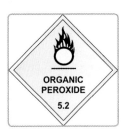

### Organic Peroxide

Chemical safety symbol used in the transport and storage of organic peroxides.

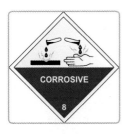

### Corrosive

The corrosive symbol is used in the transport of corrosive materials-again, avoid contact with the skin.

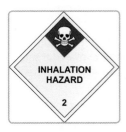

### Inhalation Hazard

Inhalation hazard transport/storage symbol.

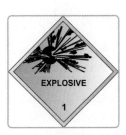

### Explosive

Used in the transport of explosive materials.

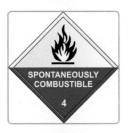

### Spontaneously Combustible

Spontaneously combustible material (treat with great caution!).

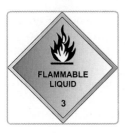

### Flammable Liquid

Used in the transport of flammable liquids.

## GENERAL SAFETY PRECAUTIONS

### Personal Safety

- Wear shoes that fully cover the feet, shoes provide a great deal of initial protection in the case of dropped containers, spilled chemicals, and unseen hazards on the floor.
- Laboratory coats or aprons must be worn over clothes. Snaps or fasteners are preferable to buttons for quicker removal in case of an emergency. Tie back long hair so that it will not fall into chemicals (Use clothes which are not too loose, especially at the sleeves).
- Gloves should be selected on the basis of the material being handled and the particular hazard involved. Glove manufacturers and the material safety data sheets (MSDSs) accompanying products in use are good sources of specific glove selection information:
  - **Polyvinyl chloride (PVC):** Protects against mild corrosives and irritants.
  - **Latex:** Provides light protection against irritants and limited protection against infectious agents.
  - **Natural rubber:** Protects against mild corrosive material and electric shock.
  - **Neoprene:** For working with solvents, oils, or mild corrosive material.
  - **Cotton:** Absorbs perspiration, keeps objects clean, and provides some limited fire retardant properties.
  - **Zetex:** When handling small burning objects. These are a good replacement for asbestos gloves. (Asbestos containing gloves may not be purchased or used in laboratories since asbestos is a known carcinogen).
- Wearing shorts and miniskirts is not allowed in the laboratory, exposed body skin give added risk to irritation and burns by corrosive chemicals and gases.
- Goggles must be worn anytime and it required to be worn, should also be worn over prescription glasses. Contact lenses should not be used during the laboratory. Goggles designed for contact wearers should be made available.
- Apron when working with dangerous chemicals, hot liquids or solids, and other potential sources of splashes, splattering or spills.
- Assume all chemicals to be poisonous either by themselves or because of impurities. Also avoid direct contact with organic chemicals since many are absorbed directly through the skin.
- If a solution, a solid or liquid chemical is spilled on the bench or on the laboratory floor, clean up the spill immediately. Any chemical spilled on the skin or clothing, should be washed immediately and thoroughly, safety officer should be notified.
- Fume hood should be used when it is indicated to do so; fume hoods remove toxic vapors and irritating odors from the laboratory. The removal of these materials is essential for protecting the health and safety of those people working in the laboratory.
- An approved safety shower and eyewash must be provided within the work area for immediate use (within 10–15 seconds of exposure) where eye hazards are present. Squirt bottle eyewashes are not acceptable in areas where corrosive chemicals are used or stored.

## Safety with Chemicals and Dissecting Specimens

- Do not touch or taste any chemical.
- Read chemical labels more than once before using the contents, it is easy to confuse chemicals.
- When working with chemicals or dissections, keep your hands away from your face. (The skin on your face is much more sensitive to irritation than your hands).
- To smell something, hold it away from your nose and wave your hand over it towards your nose.
- Flush any chemical spill on your skin with plenty of water.
- When heating anything in a test tube, the mouth of the test tube should points towards a wall, away from people.
- When mixing acids and water, acid should be poured into the water.

## CHEMICAL STORAGE

### Basic Legal Requirements

Occupational Safety and Health Administration (OSHA) has three basic legal requirements for storing chemicals: Each chemical you store must have an accompanying MSDS that lists the substance's known toxicity, flammability or acidic or caustic properties as well as how the chemical behaves in fire, an accidental exposure incident and how spills are treated; the MSDS must be readily available when needed.

- Segregate incompatible chemicals (e.g., storing oxidizing acids and flammable solvents in separate locations). This is to prevent inadvertent mixing of incompatible chemicals which can produce harmful gases/vapors, heat, fire and explosions.
- Store hazardous materials away from heat and direct sunlight. Heat and sunlight may impact and degrade chemicals, deteriorate storage containers and labels.
- Do not store hazardous materials (except cleaners) under sinks.
- Ensure caps and lids are securely tightened on containers. This prevents leaks and evaporation of contents.
- Use approved flammable storage lockers or flammable storage containers to store flammable and combustible liquids exceeding 10 gallons in one room. Flammable and combustible liquids kept in squeeze bottles and other secondary containers may be kept on counter and bench tops provided they do not exceed the 10 gallon limit and are kept in secondary containment.
- Refrigerators used for storing flammable and combustible liquids shall be designed for that purpose. Do not use ordinary domestic units.
- Label refrigerators used for storing chemicals, samples or media as follows: "Caution—Do Not Store Food or Beverages in This Refrigerator." Labels may be fabricated by users provided they are legible and securely affixed to the refrigerator.

### Chemical Storage Facilities

Chemicals need to be separated and stored by their particular class, preferably in separate cabinets. Chemicals that have a negative interaction with one another should be stored some distance apart to avoid accidentally triggering a hazardous situation. For example, solvents should be stored together in a fire-resistant cabinet while oxidizing agents should be stored well away from them. Similarly, acids such as nitric, acetic, sulfuric and hydrochloric should be gathered away from such bases as potassium and sodium hydroxides, aqueous ammonia, slaked lime and sodium carbonate. They are corrosive and when mixed with acids, can become heat-generating. Additionally, all cylinders must be labeled on the cylinder's shoulder with either the type of chemical or its trade name.

## CHEMICAL STORAGE GROUPS

Ranking chemical storage groups: From most hazardous to least hazardous
- Group 1: **Flammables**
- Group 2: **Volatile poisons**
- Group 3: **Oxidizing acids**
- Group 4: **Organic and mineral acids**
- Group 5: **Liquid bases**
- Group 6: **Liquid oxidizers**
- Group 7: **Non-volatile poisons**
- Group 8: **Metal hydrides**
- Group 9: **Dry solids.**

### Storage Group Definitions

- **Group 1: Flammable liquids:** It includes liquids with flashpoints < 100° F. Examples include all alcohols, acetone, acetaldehyde, acetonitrile, amyl acetate, benzene, cyclohexane, dimethyldichlorosilane, dioxane, ether, ethyl acetate, histoclad, hexane, hydrazine, methylbutane, picolene, piperidine, propanol, pyridine, some scintillation liquids, all silanes, tetrahydrofuran, toluene, triethylamine, and xylene.

  **Primary storage concern:** Protect flammable liquids from ignition.

  **Acceptable storage facilities/methods:**
  - Store in a flammable cabinet
  - Store in a flammable-storage refrigerator/freezer.

- **Group 2: Volatile poisons:** It includes poisons, toxics, and select and suspected carcinogens with strong odor or an evaporation rate greater than 1 (butyl acetate = 1). Examples include carbon tetrachloride, chloroform, dimethylformamide, dimethyl sulfate, formamide, formaldehyde, halothane, mercaptoethanol, methylene chloride, and phenol.

  **Primary storage concern:** Prevent volatile poison inhalation exposures.

  **Acceptable storage facilities/methods:**

    – Store in a flammable cabinet

    – Store containers of less than one liter in a refrigerator.

- **Group 3: Oxidizing acids**

  All oxidizing acids are highly reactive with most substances and each other. Examples include nitric, sulfuric, perchloric, phosphoric, and chromic acids.

  **Primary storage concern:** Prevent contact and reaction between oxidizing acids and other substances and prevent corrosive action on surfaces.

  **Acceptable storage facilities/methods:**
  – Store in a safety cabinet
  – Each oxidizing acid must be double-contained (i.e., the primary container must be kept inside a canister, tray or tub).

- **Group 4: Organic and mineral acids**

  **Organic and mineral acids.** Examples include acetic, butyric, formic, glacial acetic, hydrochloric, isobutyric, mercaptoproprionic, proprionic, and trifluoroacetic acids.

  **Primary storage concern:** Prevent contact and reaction with bases and oxidizing acids and prevent corrosive action on surfaces.

  **Acceptable storage facilities/methods:**
  – Store in a safety cabinet.

- **Group 5: Liquid bases**

  **Liquid bases.** Examples include sodium hydroxide, ammonium hydroxide, calcium hydroxide, and gluteraldehyde.

  **Primary storage concern:** Prevent contact and reaction with acids.

  **Acceptable storage facilities/methods:**
  – In a safety cabinet
  – In tubs or trays in normal cabinet.

**Compatible storage groups:** Liquid bases may be stored with flammables in the flammable cabinet if volatile poisons are not stored there.

- **Group 6: Liquid oxidizers**

  Oxidizing liquids react with everything, potentially causing explosions or corrosion of surfaces. Examples include ammonium persulfate and hydrogen peroxide (if greater than or equal to 30%).

  **Primary storage concern:** Isolate liquid oxidizers from other substances.

  **Acceptable storage facilities/methods:**
  – Total quantities exceeding three liters must be kept in a cabinet housing no other chemicals.
  – Smaller quantities must be double-contained when stored near other chemicals (e.g. in a refrigerator).

- **Group 7: Non-volatile liquid poisons**

  It includes highly toxic (LD50 oral rat < 50 mg/kg) and toxic chemicals (LD50 oral rat < 500 mg/kg), select carcinogens, suspected carcinogens, and mutagens. Examples include acrylamide solutions, coomassie blue stain, diethylpyrocarbonate, diisopropyl fluorophosphate, uncured epoxy resins, ethidium bromide, and triethanolamine.

  **Primary storage concern:** Prevent contact and reaction between non-volatile liquid poisons and other substances.

  **Acceptable storage facilities/methods:**
  - Store in a cabinet or refrigerator (i.e., non-volatile liquid poisons must be enclosed)
  - Do not store on open shelves in the laboratory or cold room.
  - Liquid poisons in containers larger than one liter must be stored below bench level on shelves closest to the floor. Smaller containers of liquid poison can be stored above bench level only if behind sliding (non-swinging) doors.

- **Group 8: Metal hydrides**

  Most metal hydrides react violently with water, some ignite spontaneously in air (pyrophoric). Examples include sodium borohydride, calcium hydride, and lithium aluminum hydride.

  **Primary storage concern:** Prevent contact and reaction with liquids and, in some cases, air.

  **Acceptable storage facilities/methods:**
  - Store using secure, waterproof double-containment according to label instructions
  - Isolate from other storage groups.

- **Group 9: Dry solids**

  **It includes all powders, hazardous and non-hazardous.** Examples include benzidine, cyanogen bromide, ethylmaleimide, oxalic acid, potassium cyanide, and sodium cyanide.

  **Primary storage concern:** Prevent contact and potential reaction with liquids.

  **Acceptable storage facilities/methods:**
  - Cabinets are recommended, but if not available, open shelves are acceptable.
- Store above liquids
- Warning labels on highly toxic powders should be inspected and highlighted or ended to stand out against less toxic substances in this group.
- It is recommended that the most hazardous substances in this group be segregated.
- It is particularly important to keep liquid poisons below cyanide-containing or sulfide-containing poisons (solids); a spill of aqueous liquid onto cyanide-containing or sulfide-containing poisons would cause a reaction that would release poisonous gas.

## Storage Recommendations

- Hazardous materials are often transferred to squeeze bottles and other plastic containers such as Nalgene bottles. These are made of plastics, such as high-density polyethylene, low-density polyethylene and polypropylene and may exhibit varying degrees of resistance to different chemicals. Moreover, they may deteriorate over time, especially when exposed to sunlight or UV sources.
- Secondary containment for Liquids, store liquid hazardous materials (including squeeze and wash bottles) in secondary containment. This is to minimize the impact and spread of spills resulting from broken/leaking containers. Secondary containment capacity must be 110% of the largest container or 10% of the aggregate volume of all containers, whichever is larger.
- Conduct periodic cleanouts to minimize accumulating unwanted chemicals.

## Chemical Inventory

Inventories of reagents are essential in the control of chemical hazards. They enable the staff to determine the existence of a specific reagent chemical, its location, and its approximate shelf age. A reagent chemical inventory should be conducted at least once a year. The chemical inventory record should:

- Contain the date the inventory was conducted
- Identify chemical reagents by name and formula
- Specify the amount of each reagent present
- Indicate the storage location of each reagent
- Indicate the hazard of each reagent, using information from the material data safety sheet (MSDS) for each substance and the appropriate National Fire Protection Association hazard code
- Indicate the arrival date and quantity of all reagents received.

## Safeguard Against Theft

To prevent theft, laboratory workers should make sure that laboratory doors are locked when unattended.

## Chemical Spills in the Laboratory

In all cases, immediately alert safety officer of the spill, the following equipment should also be provided:

1. Chemical spill kits
2. Protective clothing, e.g. heavy-duty rubber gloves, overshoes or rubber boots and respirators
3. Scoops and dustpans
4. Forceps for picking up broken glass
5. Mops, cloths and paper towels
6. Buckets
7. Soda ash (sodium carbonate, $Na_2CO_3$) or sodium bicarbonate ($NaHCO_3$) for neutralizing acids and corrosive chemicals

8. Sand (to cover alkali spills)
9. Non-flammable detergent.

### The Following Actions should be Taken in the Event of a Significant Chemical Spill

1. Notify the appropriate safety officer
2. Evacuate non-essential personnel from the area
3. Attend to persons who may have been contaminated
4. If the spilled material is flammable, extinguish all open flames, turn-off gas in the room and adjacent areas, open windows (if possible), and switch off electrical equipment that may spark.
5. Avoid breathing vapor from spilled material.
6. Establish exhaust ventilation if it is safe to do so.
7. Secure the necessary items (see above) to clean up the spill.

- **Non-volatile and non-flammable materials:** If the material is not particularly volatile, nor toxic, and poses no fire hazard the liquid can be cleaned up by using an absorbent material which neutralizes them, for example, sodium bicarbonate solution or powder for acids, or sodium thiosulfate solution for bromine. Rubber or plastic gloves should be worn while using absorbent materials. A dustpan and brush should be used to remove the absorbent material. Then, the contaminated area should be cleaned with detergent and water and the area mopped dry.

- **Acid spills:** Apply neutralizer (or sodium bicarbonate) to perimeter of spill. Mix thoroughly until fizzing and evolution of gas ceases.

  NOTE: It may be necessary to add water to the mixture to complete the reaction. Neutralizer has a tendency to absorb acid before fully neutralizing it. Check mixture with pH indicator paper to assure that the acid has been neutralized. Transfer the mixture to a plastic bag, tie shut, fill out a waste label, and place in the fume hood.

- **Caustic spills:** Apply neutralizer to perimeter of spill. Mix thoroughly until fizzing and evolution of gas ceases. Check mixture with pH indicator paper to assure that the material has been completely neutralized. Transfer the mixture to a plastic bag, tie shut, fill out a waste label, and place in the fume hood.

- **Solvent spills:** Apply activated charcoal to the perimeter of the spill. Mix thoroughly until material is dry and no evidence of liquid solvent remains. Transfer absorbed solvent to a plastic bag (if compatible), tie shut, and fill out and attach a waste label, and place in the fume hood.

- **Mercury Spills:** Using a mercury vacuum, vacuum all areas where mercury was spilled with particular attention to corners, cracks, depressions and creases in flooring or table tops. To clean up small spills with a mercury spill kit, dampen the mercury sponge with water, then wipe the contaminated area. Do this procedure slowly to allow for complete absorption of all free mercury. A silvery surface will form on the sponge. Place the contaminated sponge in its plastic bag, tie shut, fill out and attach a waste label, and place in the fume hood.

## Chemical Spills on a Person

- **Over the body:** Within seconds, quickly remove all contaminated clothing while person is under safety shower. Flood the affected body area with cold water for at least fifteen minutes. If pain continues or resumes, flood with more water. Wash off chemicals with a mild detergent solution. Do not apply any materials such as neutralizing agents or salves, to the area. Obtain medical assistance immediately.

- **On small area of body:** Immediately flush area thoroughly with cold water. Wash with a mild detergent solution. If there is no visible burn, wash out the area with warm water and soap.

- **In the eyes:** You will need to assist the person who has chemicals spattered in the eyes. Immediately drench the eyes at the nearest emergency eyewash station. Force the eye or eyes open to get water into them. The speed of your response to this emergency is extremely important. Notify the laboratory instructor of the accident immediately.

## Swallowing Chemicals

The laboratory safety officer should determine what specific substance is ingested. The individual should be forced to drink copious amounts of water while en route to medical assistance. The Health Center or Hospital should be notified while the individual is in transit as to what chemicals are involved.

## Material Safety Data Sheets

Material safety data sheets (MSDSs), are designed to provide the information needed to protect users from any hazards that may be associated with the product. MSDSs have become the primary vehicle through which the potential hazards of materials obtained from commercial sources are communicated to the laboratory worker. Institutions are required to retain and make readily available to workers the MSDSs provided by chemical suppliers.

As the first step in a risk-assessment, laboratory workers should examine their plan for a proposed experiment and identify the chemicals whose toxicological properties they are not already familiar with from previous experience. The MSDS for each unfamiliar chemical should then be examined. Procedures for accessing MSDS files vary from institution to institution. In some cases, MSDS files may be present in each laboratory, while in many cases complete files of MSDSs are maintained only in a central location, some laboratories have the capability to access MSDSs electronically, either from CD-ROM disks or via computer networks. As a last resort, the laboratory worker can always contact the chemical supplier directly and request that an MSDS be sent by mail. MSDSs are concise technical documents, generally two to five pages in length. An MSDS typically begins with a compilation of data on the physical, chemical, and toxicological properties of the substance and then provides generally concise suggestions for handling, storage, and disposal. Finally, emergency and first-aid procedures are usually outlined. At present, there is no required format for an MSDS.

## Immediately Dangerous to Life and Health

This section lists the immediately dangerous chemicals to life or health concentrations (IDLHs). These criteria formed a tiered approach, preferentially using acute human toxicity data, followed by acute animal inhalation toxicity data, and then by acute animal oral toxicity data to determine a preliminary updated IDLH value. When relevant acute toxicity data were insufficient or unavailable, chronic toxicity data or an analogy to a chemically similar substance is considered.

The purpose for establishing an IDLH value to determine the airborne concentration from which a staff could escape without injury or irreversible health effects from an IDLH exposure in the event of the failure of respiratory protection equipment. The IDLH was considered a maximum concentration above which only a highly reliable breathing apparatus providing maximum worker protection should be permitted. In determining IDLH values, it is considered the ability of a staff to escape without loss of life or irreversible health effects along with certain transient effects, such as severe eye or respiratory irritation, disorientation, and incoordination, which could prevent escape. As a safety margin, IDLH values are based on effects that might occur as a consequence of a 30-minute exposure. However, the 30-minute period was not meant to imply that staffs should stay in the work environment any longer than necessary; in fact, every effort should be made to exit immediately (Table 2.2).

## Transport

The most widely applied regulatory scheme is that for the transportation of dangerous goods. The United Nations Economic and Social Council issues

**Table 2.2** Chemical listing and documentation of IDLH values

| Substance | Original IDLH value | Revised IDLH value |
|---|---|---|
| Acetaldehyde | 10,000 ppm | 2,000 ppm |
| Acetic acid | 1,000 ppm | 50 ppm |
| Acetic anhydride | 1,000 ppm | 200 ppm |
| Acetone | 20,000 ppm | 2,500 ppm [LEL] |
| Acetonitrile | 4,000 ppm | 500 ppm |
| Acetylene tetrabromide | 10 ppm | 8 ppm |
| Acrolein | 5 ppm | 2 ppm |
| Acrylamide | Unknown | 60 mg/m$^3$ |
| Acrylonitrile | 500 ppm | 85 ppm |
| Aldrin | 100 mg/m$^3$ | 25 mg/m$^3$ |
| Allyl alcohol | 150 ppm | 20 ppm |
| Allyl chloride | 300 ppm | 250 ppm |
| Allyl glycidyl ether | 270 ppm | 50 ppm |
| 2 aminopyridine | 5 ppm | 5 ppm [Unch] |
| Ammonia | 500 ppm | 300 ppm |

*Contd...*

Contd...

| Substance | Original IDLH value | Revised IDLH value |
|---|---|---|
| Ammonium sulfamate | 5,000 mg/m³ | 1,500 mg/m³ |
| n-amyl acetate | 4,000 ppm | 1,000 ppm |
| sec-Amyl acetate | 9,000 ppm | 1,000 ppm |
| Aniline | 100 ppm | 100 ppm [Unch] |
| o-Anisidine | 50 mg/m³ | 50 mg/m³ [Unch] |
| p-Anisidine | 50 mg/m³ | 50 mg/m³ [Unch] |
| Antimony compounds (as Sb) | 80 mg Sb/m³ | 50 mg Sb/m³ |
| ANTU | 100 mg/m³ | 100 mg/m³ [Unch] |
| Arsenic (inorganic compounds, as As) | 100 mg As/m³ | 5 mg As/m³ |
| Arsine | 6 ppm | 3 ppm |
| Azinphosmethyl | 20 mg/m³ | 10 mg/m³ |
| Barium (soluble compounds, as Ba) | 1,100 mg Ba/m³ | 50 mg Ba/m³ |
| Benzene | 3,000 ppm | 500 ppm |
| Benzoyl peroxide | 7,000 mg/m³ | 1,500 mg/m³ |
| Benzyl chloride | 10 ppm | 10 ppm [Unch] |
| Beryllium compounds (as Be) | 10 mg Be/m³ | 4 mg Be/m³ |
| Boron oxide | No evidence | 2,000 mg/m³ |
| Boron trifluoride | 100 ppm | 25 ppm |
| Bromine | 10 ppm | 3 ppm |
| Bromoform | Unknown | 850 ppm |
| 1,3-Butadiene | 20,000 ppm [LEL] | 2,000 ppm [LEL] |
| 2-Butanone | 3,000 ppm | 3,000 ppm [Unch] |
| 2-Butoxyethanol | 700 ppm | 700 ppm [Unch] |
| n-Butyl acetate | 10,000 ppm | 1,700 ppm [LEL] |
| sec-Butyl acetate | 10,000 ppm | 1,700 ppm [LEL] |
| tert-Butyl acetate | 10,000 ppm | 1,500 ppm [LEL] |
| n-Butyl alcohol | 8,000 ppm | 1,400 ppm [LEL] |
| sec-Butyl alcohol | 10,000 ppm | 2,000 ppm |
| tert-Butyl alcohol | 8,000 ppm | 1,600 ppm |
| n-Butylamine | 2,000 ppm | 300 ppm |
| tert-Butyl chromate | 30 mg/m³ (as CrO3) | 15 mg Cr(VI)/m³ |
| n-Butyl glycidyl ether | 3,500 ppm | 250 ppm |
| n-Butyl mercaptan | 2,500 ppm | 500 ppm |
| p-tert-Butyltoluene | 1,000 ppm | 100 ppm |
| Cadmium dust (as Cd) | 50 mg Cd/m³ | 9 mg Cd/m³ |
| Cadmium fume (as Cd) | 9 mg Cd/m³ | 9 mg Cd/m³[Unch] |
| Calcium arsenate (as As) | 100 mg As/m³ | 5 mg As/m³ |

Contd...

Contd...

| Substance | Original IDLH value | Revised IDLH value |
|---|---|---|
| Camphor (synthetic) | 200 mg/m³ | 200 mg/m³ [Unch] |
| Carbaryl | 600 mg/m³ | 100 mg/m³ |
| Carbon black | No evidence | 1,750 mg/m³ |
| Carbon dioxide | 50,000 ppm | 40,000 ppm |
| Carbon disulfide | 500 ppm | 500 ppm [Unch] |
| Carbon monoxide | 1,500 ppm | 1,200 ppm |
| Carbon tetrachloride | 300 ppm | 200 ppm |
| Chlordane | 500 mg/m³ | 100 mg/m³ |
| Chlorinated camphene | 200 mg/m³ | 200 mg/m³ [Unch] |
| Chlorinated diphenyl oxide | Unknown | 5 mg/m³ |
| Chlorine | 30 ppm | 10 ppm |
| Chlorine dioxide | 10 ppm | 5 ppm |
| Chlorine trifluoride | 20 ppm | 20 ppm [Unch] |
| Chloroacetaldehyde | 100 ppm | 45 ppm |
| α-Chloroacetophenone | 100 mg/m³ | 15 mg/m³ |
| Chlorobenzene | 2,400 ppm | 1,000 ppm |
| o-Chlorobenzylidene malononitrile | 2 mg/m³ | 2 mg/m³ [Unch] |
| Chlorobromomethane | 5,000 ppm | 2,000 ppm |
| Chlorodiphenyl (42% chlorine) | 10 mg/m³ | 5 mg/m³ |
| Chlorodiphenyl (54% chlorine) | 5 mg/m³ | 5 mg/m³ [Unch] |
| Chloroform | 1,000 ppm | 500 ppm |
| 1-Chloro-1-nitropropane | 2,000 ppm | 100 ppm |
| Chloropicrin | 4 ppm | 2 ppm |
| β-Chloroprene | 400 ppm | 300 ppm |
| Chromic acid and chromates | 30 mg/m³ (as CrO3) | 15 mg Cr(VI)/m³ |
| Chromium (II) compounds [as Cr(II)] | No evidence | 250 mg Cr(II)/m³ |
| Chromium (III) compounds [as Cr(III)] | No evidence | 25 mg Cr(III)/m³ |
| Chromium metal (as Cr) | No evidence | 250 mg Cr/m³ |
| Coal tar pitch volatiles | 700 mg/m³ | 80 mg/m³ |
| Cobalt metal, dust and fume (as Co) | 20 mg Co/m³ | 20 mg Co/m³ [Unch] |
| Copper (dusts and mists, as Cu) | No evidence | 100 mg Cu/m³ |
| Copper fume (as Cu) | No evidence | 100 mg Cu/m³ |
| Cotton dust (raw) | No evidence | 100 mg/m³ |
| Crag (r) herbicide | 5,000 mg/m³ | 500 mg/m³ |
| Cresol (o, m, p isomers) | 250 ppm | 250 ppm [Unch] |
| Crotonaldehyde | 400 ppm | 50 ppm |

Contd...

*Contd...*

| Substance | Original IDLH value | Revised IDLH value |
|---|---|---|
| Cumene | 8,000 ppm | 900 ppm [LEL] |
| Cyanides (as CN) | 50 mg/m³ (as CN) | 25 mg/m³ (as CN) |
| Cyclohexane | 10,000 ppm | 1,300 ppm [LEL] |
| Cyclohexanol | 3,500 ppm | 400 ppm |
| Cyclohexanone | 5,000 ppm | 700 ppm |
| Cyclohexene | 10,000 ppm | 2,000 ppm |
| Cyclopentadiene | 2,000 ppm | 750 ppm |
| 2,4-D | 500 mg/m³ | 100 mg/m³ |
| Dichloro-diphenyl-tricholoroethane | No evidence | 500 mg/m³ |
| Decaborane | 100 mg/m³ | 15 mg/m³ |
| Demeton | 20 mg/m³ | 10 mg/m³ |
| Diacetone alcohol | 2,100 ppm | 1,800 ppm [LEL] |
| Diazomethane | 2 ppm | 2 ppm [Unch] |
| Diborane | 40 ppm | 15 ppm |
| Dibutyl phosphate | 125 ppm | 30 ppm |
| Dibutyl phthalate | 9,300 mg/m³ | 4,000 mg/m³ |
| o-Dichlorobenzene | 1,000 ppm | 200 ppm |
| p-Dichlorobenzene | 1,000 ppm | 150 ppm |
| Dichlorodifluoromethane | 50,000 ppm | 15,000 ppm |
| 1,3-Dichloro 5,5-dimethylhydantoin | Unknown | 5 mg/m³ |
| 1,1-Dichloroethane | 4,000 ppm | 3,000 ppm |
| 1,2-Dichloroethylene | 4,000 ppm | 1,000 ppm |
| Dichloroethyl ether | 250 ppm | 100 ppm |
| Dichloromonofluoromethane | 50,000 ppm | 5,000 ppm |
| 1,1-Dichloro 1-nitroethane | 150 ppm | 25 ppm |
| Dichlorotetrafluoroethane | 50,000 ppm | 15,000 ppm |
| Dichlorvos | 200 mg/m³ | 100 mg/m³ |
| Dieldrin | 450 mg/m³ | 50 mg/m³ |
| Diethylamine | 2,000 ppm | 200 ppm |
| 2-Diethylaminoethanol | 500 ppm | 100 ppm |
| Difluorodibromomethane | 2,500 ppm | 2,000 ppm |
| Diglycidyl ether | 25 ppm | 10 ppm |
| Diisobutyl ketone | 2,000 ppm | 500 ppm |
| Diisopropylamine | 1,000 ppm | 200 ppm |
| Dimethyl acetamide | 400 ppm | 300 ppm |
| Dimethylamine | 2,000 ppm | 500 ppm |
| N,N-Dimethylaniline | 100 ppm | 100 ppm [Unch] |

*Contd...*

*Contd...*

| Substance | Original IDLH value | Revised IDLH value |
|---|---|---|
| Dimethyl 1,2-dibromo 2,2-dichlorethyl phosphate | 1,800 mg/m³ | 200 mg/m³ |
| Dimethylformamide | 3,500 ppm | 500 ppm |
| 1,1-Dimethylhydrazine | 50 ppm | 15 ppm |
| Dimethylphthalate | 9,300 mg/m³ | 2,000 mg/m³ |
| Dimethyl sulfate | 10 ppm | 7 ppm |
| Dinitrobenzene (o, m, p isomers) | 200 mg/m³ | 50 mg/m³ |
| Dinitroocresol | 5 mg/m³ | 5 mg/m³ [Unch] |
| Dinitrotoluene | 200 mg/m³ | 50 mg/m³ |
| Di sec-octyl phthalate | Unknown | 5,000 mg/m³ |
| Dioxane | 2,000 ppm | 500 ppm |
| Diphenyl | 300 mg/m³ | 100 mg/m³ |
| Dipropylene glycol methyl ether | Unknown | 600 ppm |
| Endrin | 2,000 mg/m³ | 2 mg/m³ |
| Epichlorohydrin | 250 ppm | 75 ppm |
| Ethylp-nitrophenyl phenylphosphorothioate | 50 mg/m³ | 5 mg/m³ |
| Ethanolamine | 1,000 ppm | 30 ppm |
| 2-Ethoxyethanol | 6,000 ppm | 500 ppm |
| 2-Ethoxyethyl acetate | 2,500 ppm | 500 ppm |
| Ethyl acetate | 10,000 ppm | 2,000 ppm [LEL] |
| Ethyl acrylate | 2,000 ppm | 300 ppm |
| Ethyl alcohol | 15,000 ppm | 3,300 ppm [LEL] |
| Ethylamine | 4,000 ppm | 600 ppm |
| Ethyl benzene | 2,000 ppm | 800 ppm [LEL] |
| Ethyl bromide | 3,500 ppm | 2,000 ppm |
| Ethyl butyl ketone | 3,000 ppm | 1,000 ppm |
| Ethyl chloride | 20,000 ppm | 3,800 ppm [LEL] |
| Ethylene chlorohydrin | 10 ppm | 7 ppm |
| Ethylenediamine | 2,000 ppm | 1,000 ppm |
| Ethylene dibromide | 400 ppm | 100 ppm |
| Ethylene dichloride | 1,000 ppm | 50 ppm |
| Ethylene glycol dinitrate | 500 mg/m³ | 75 mg/m³ |
| Ethyleneimine | 100 ppm | 100 ppm [Unch] |
| Ethylene oxide | 800 ppm | 800 ppm [Unch] |
| Ethyl ether | 19,000 ppm [LEL] | 1,900 ppm [LEL] |
| Ethyl formate | 8,000 ppm | 1,500 ppm |
| Ethyl mercaptan | 2,500 ppm | 500 ppm |

*Contd...*

*Contd...*

| Substance | Original IDLH value | Revised IDLH value |
|---|---|---|
| N-Ethylmorpholine | 2,000 ppm | 100 ppm |
| Ethyl silicate | 1,000 ppm | 700 ppm |
| Ferbam | No evidence | 800 mg/m³ |
| Ferrovanadium dust | No evidence | 500 mg/m³ |
| Fluorides (as F) | 500 mg F/m³ | 250 mg F/m³ |
| Fluorine | 25 ppm | 25 ppm [Unch] |
| Fluorotrichloromethane | 10,000 ppm | 2,000 ppm |
| Formaldehyde | 30 ppm | 20 ppm |
| Formic acid | 30 ppm | 30 ppm [Unch] |
| Furfural | 250 ppm | 100 ppm |
| Furfuryl alcohol | 250 ppm | 75 ppm |
| Glycidol | 500 ppm | 150 ppm |
| Graphite (natural) | No evidence | 1,250 mg/m³ |
| Hafnium compounds (as Hf) | Unknown | 50 mg Hf/m³ |
| Heptachlor | 700 mg/m³ | 35 mg/m³ |
| n-Heptane | 5,000 ppm | 750 ppm |
| Hexachloroethane | 300 ppm | 300 ppm [Unch] |
| Hexachloronaphthalene | 2 mg/m³ | 2 mg/m³ [Unch] |
| n-Hexane | 5,000 ppm | 1,100 ppm [LEL] |
| 2-Hexanone | 5,000 ppm | 1,600 ppm |
| Hexone | 3,000 ppm | 500 ppm |
| sec-Hexyl acetate | 4,000 ppm | 500 ppm |
| Hydrazine | 80 ppm | 50 ppm |
| Hydrogen bromide | 50 ppm | 30 ppm |
| Hydrogen chloride | 100 ppm | 50 ppm |
| Hydrogen cyanide | 50 ppm | 50 ppm [Unch] |
| Hydrogen fluoride (as F) | 30 ppm | 30 ppm [Unch] |
| Hydrogen peroxide | 75 ppm | 75 ppm [Unch] |
| Hydrogen selenide (as Se) | 2 ppm | 1 ppm |
| Hydrogen sulfide | 300 ppm | 100 ppm |
| Hydroquinone | Unknown | 50 mg/m³ |
| Iodine | 10 ppm | 2 ppm |
| Iron oxide dust and fume (as Fe) | No evidence | 2,500 mg Fe/m³ |
| Isoamyl acetate | 3,000 ppm | 1,000 ppm |
| Isoamyl alcohol (primary and secondary) | 10,000 ppm | 500 ppm |
| Isobutyl acetate | 7,500 ppm | 1,300 ppm [LEL] |
| Isobutyl alcohol | 8,000 ppm | 1,600 ppm |

*Contd...*

*Contd...*

| Substance | Original IDLH value | Revised IDLH value |
|---|---|---|
| Isophorone | 800 ppm | 200 ppm |
| Isopropyl acetate | 16,000 ppm | 1,800 ppm |
| Isopropyl alcohol | 12,000 ppm | 2,000 ppm [LEL] |
| Isopropylamine | 4,000 ppm | 750 ppm |
| Isopropyl ether | 10,000 ppm | 1,400 ppm [LEL] |
| Isopropyl glycidyl ether | 1,000 ppm | 400 ppm |
| Ketene | Unknown | 5 ppm |
| Lead compounds (as Pb) | 700 mg Pb/m$^3$ | 100 mg Pb/m$^3$ |
| Lindane | 1,000 mg/m$^3$ | 50 mg/m$^3$ |
| Lithium hydride | 55 mg/m$^3$ | 0.5 mg/m$^3$ |
| Liquefied petroleum gas | 19,000 ppm [LEL] | 2,000 ppm [LEL] |
| Magnesium oxide fume | No evidence | 750 mg/m$^3$ |
| Malathion | 5,000 mg/m$^3$ | 250 mg/m$^3$ |
| Maleic anhydride | Unknown | 10 mg/m$^3$ |
| Manganese compounds (as Mn) | No evidence | 500 mg Mn/m$^3$ |
| Mercury compounds [except (organo) alkyls, as Hg] | 28 mg Hg/m$^3$ | 10 mg Hg/m$^3$ |
| Mercury (organo) alkyl compounds (as Hg) | 10 mg Hg/m$^3$ | 2 mg Hg/m$^3$ |
| Mesityl oxide | 5,000 ppm | 1,400 ppm [LEL] |
| Methoxychlor | No evidence | 5,000 mg/m$^3$ |
| Methyl acetate | 10,000 ppm | 3,100 ppm [LEL] |
| Methyl acetylene | 15,000 ppm [LEL] | 1,700 ppm [LEL] |
| Methyl acetylenepropadiene mixture | 15,000 ppm | 3,400 ppm [LEL] |
| Methyl acrylate | 1,000 ppm | 250 ppm |
| Methylal | 15,000 ppm [LEL] | 2,200 ppm [LEL] |
| Methyl alcohol | 25,000 ppm | 6,000 ppm |
| Methylamine | 100 ppm | 100 ppm [Unch] |
| Methyl (namyl) ketone | 4,000 ppm | 800 ppm |
| Methyl bromide | 2,000 ppm | 250 ppm |
| Methyl cellosolve (r) | 2,000 ppm | 200 ppm |
| Methyl cellosolve (r) acetate | 4,000 ppm | 200 ppm |
| Methyl chloride | 10,000 ppm | 2,000 ppm |
| Methyl chloroform | 1,000 ppm | 700 ppm |
| Methylcyclohexane | 10,000 ppm | 1,200 ppm [LEL] |
| Methylcyclohexanol | 10,000 ppm | 500 ppm |
| o-Methylcyclohexanone | 2,500 ppm | 600 ppm |
| Methylene bisphenyl isocyanate | 100 mg/m$^3$ | 75 mg/m$^3$ |

*Contd...*

*Contd...*

| Substance | Original IDLH value | Revised IDLH value |
|---|---|---|
| Methylene chloride | 5,000 ppm | 2,300 ppm |
| Methyl formate | 5,000 ppm | 4,500 ppm |
| 5-Methyl 3-heptanone | 3,000 ppm | 100 ppm |
| Methyl hydrazine | 50 ppm | 20 ppm |
| Methyl iodide | 800 ppm | 100 ppm |
| Methyl isobutyl carbinol | 2,000 ppm | 400 ppm |
| Methyl isocyanate | 20 ppm | 3 ppm |
| Methyl mercaptan | 400 ppm | 150 ppm |
| Methyl methacrylate | 4,000 ppm | 1,000 ppm |
| Methyl styrene | 5,000 ppm | 700 ppm |
| Mica | No evidence | 1,500 mg/m$^3$ |
| Molybdenum (insoluble compounds, as Mo) | No evidence | 5,000 mg Mo/m$^3$ |
| Molybdenum (soluble compounds, as Mo) | No evidence | 1,000 mg Mo/m$^3$ |
| Monomethyl aniline | 100 ppm | 100 ppm [Unch] |
| Morpholine | 8,000 ppm | 1,400 ppm [LEL] |
| Naphtha (coal tar) | 10,000 ppm [LEL] | 1,000 ppm [LEL] |
| Naphthalene | 500 ppm | 250 ppm |
| Nickel carbonyl (as Ni) | 7 ppm | 2 ppm |
| Nickel metal and other compounds (as Ni) | No evidence | 10 mg Ni/m$^3$ |
| Nicotine | 35 mg/m$^3$ | 5 mg/m$^3$ |
| Nitric acid | 100 ppm | 25 ppm |
| Nitric oxide | 100 ppm | 100 ppm [Unch] |
| p-Nitroaniline | 300 mg/m$^3$ | 300 mg/m$^3$ [Unch] |
| Nitrobenzene | 200 ppm | 200 ppm [Unch] |
| p-Nitrochlorobenzene | 1,000 mg/m$^3$ | 100 mg/m$^3$ |
| Nitroethane | 1,000 ppm | 1,000 ppm [Unch] |
| Nitrogen dioxide | 50 ppm | 20 ppm |
| Nitrogen trifluoride | 2,000 ppm | 1,000 ppm |
| Nitroglycerine | 500 mg/m$^3$ | 75 mg/m$^3$ |
| Nitromethane | 1,000 ppm | 750 ppm |
| 1-Nitropropane | 2,300 ppm | 1,000 ppm |
| 2-Nitropropane | 2,300 ppm | 100 ppm |
| Nitrotoluene (o, m, p isomers) | 200 ppm | 200 ppm [Unch] |
| Octachloronaphthalene | Unknown | Unknown [Unch] |
| Octane | 5,000 ppm | 1,000 ppm [LEL] |
| Oil mist (mineral) | No evidence | 2,500 mg/m$^3$ |
| Osmium tetroxide (as Os) | 1 mg Os/m$^3$ | 1 mg Os/m$^3$ [Unch] |

*Contd...*

*Contd...*

| Substance | Original IDLH value | Revised IDLH value |
|---|---|---|
| Oxalic acid | 500 mg/m³ | 500 mg/m³ [Unch] |
| Oxygen difluoride | 0.5 ppm | 0.5 ppm [Unch] |
| Ozone | 10 ppm | 5 ppm |
| Paraquat | 1.5 mg/m³ | 1 mg/m³ |
| Parathion | 20 mg/m³ | 10 mg/m³ |
| Pentaborane | 3 ppm | 1 ppm |
| Pentachloronaphthalene | Unknown | Unknown [Unch] |
| Pentachlorophenol | 150 mg/m³ | 2.5 mg/m³ |
| n-Pentane | 15,000 ppm [LEL] | 1,500 ppm [LEL] |
| 2-Pentanone | 5,000 ppm | 1,500 ppm |
| Perchloromethyl mercaptan | 10 ppm | 10 ppm [Unch] |
| Perchloryl fluoride | 385 ppm | 100 ppm |
| Petroleum distillates (naphtha) | 10,000 ppm | 1,100 ppm [LEL] |
| Phenol | 250 ppm | 250 ppm [Unch] |
| p-Phenylene diamine | Unknown | 25 mg/m³ |
| Phenyl ether (vapor) | No evidence | 100 ppm |
| Phenyl etherbiphenyl mixture (vapor) | No evidence | 10 ppm |
| Phenyl glycidyl ether | Unknown | 100 ppm |
| Phenylhydrazine | 295 ppm | 15 ppm |
| Phosdrin | 4 ppm | 4 ppm [Unch] |
| Phosgene | 2 ppm | 2 ppm [Unch] |
| Phosphine | 200 ppm | 50 ppm |
| Phosphoric acid | 10,000 mg/m³ | 1,000 mg/m³ |
| Phosphorus (yellow) | No evidence | 5 mg/m³ |
| Phosphorus pentachloride | 200 mg/m³ | 70 mg/m³ |
| Phosphorus pentasulfide | 750 mg/m³ | 250 mg/m³ |
| Phosphorus trichloride | 50 ppm | 25 ppm |
| Phthalic anhydride | 10,000 mg/m³ | 60 mg/m³ |
| Picric acid | 100 mg/m³ | 75 mg/m³ |
| Pindone | 200 mg/m³ | 100 mg/m³ |
| Platinum (soluble salts, as Pt) | No evidence | 4 mg Pt/m³ |
| Portland cement | No evidence | 5,000 mg/m³ |
| Propane | 20,000 ppm [LEL] | 2,100 ppm [LEL] |
| n-Propyl acetate | 8,000 ppm | 1,700 ppm |
| n-Propyl alcohol | 4,000 ppm | 800 ppm |
| Propylene dichloride | 2,000 ppm | 400 ppm |
| Propyleneimine | 500 ppm | 100 ppm |

*Contd...*

*Contd...*

| Substance | Original IDLH value | Revised IDLH value |
|---|---|---|
| Propylene oxide | 2,000 ppm | 400 ppm |
| n-Propyl nitrate | 2,000 ppm | 500 ppm |
| Pyrethrum | 5,000 mg/m³ | 5,000 mg/m³ [Unch] |
| Pyridine | 3,600 ppm | 1,000 ppm |
| Quinone | 300 mg/m³ | 100 mg/m³ |
| Rhodium (metal fume and insoluble compounds, as Rh) | No evidence | 100 mg Rh/m³ |
| Rhodium (soluble compounds, as Rh) | No evidence | 2 mg Rh/m³ |
| Ronnel | 5,000 mg/m³ | 300 mg/m³ |
| Rotenone | Unknown | 2,500 mg/m³ |
| Selenium compounds (as Se) | Unknown | 1 mg Se/m³ |
| Selenium hexafluoride | 5 ppm | 2 ppm |
| Silica, amorphous | No evidence | 3,000 mg/m³ |
| Silica, crystalline (respirable dust) | No evidence | |
|    cristobalite/tridymite | | 25 mg/m³ |
|    quartz/tripoli | | 50 mg/m³ |
| Silver (metal dust and soluble compounds, as Ag) | No evidence | 10 mg Ag/m³ |
| Soapstone | No evidence | 3,000 mg/m³ |
| Sodium fluoroacetate | 5 mg/m³ | 2.5 mg/m³ |
| Sodium hydroxide | 250 mg/m³ | 10 mg/m³ |
| Stibine | 40 ppm | 5 ppm |
| Stoddard solvent | 29,500 mg/m³ | 20,000 mg/m³ |
| Strychnine | 3 mg/m³ | 3 mg/m³ [Unch] |
| Styrene | 5,000 ppm | 700 ppm |
| Sulfur dioxide | 100 ppm | 100 ppm [Unch] |
| Sulfuric acid | 80 mg/m³ | 15 mg/m³ |
| Sulfur monochloride | 10 ppm | 5 ppm |
| Sulfur pentafluoride | 1 ppm | 1 ppm [Unch] |
| Sulfuryl fluoride | 1,000 ppm | 200 ppm |
| 2,4,5-T | Unknown | 250 mg/m³ |
| Talc | No evidence | 1,000 mg/m³ |
| Tantalum (metal and oxide dust, as Ta) | No evidence | 2,500 mg Ta/m³ |
| Tetraethyl dithionopyrophosphate | 35 mg/m³ | 10 mg/m³ |
| Tellurium compounds (as Te) | No evidence | 25 mg Te/m³ |
| Tellurium hexafluoride | 1 ppm | 1 ppm [Unch] |
| Tetraethyl pyrophosphate | 10 mg/m³ | 5 mg/m³ |

*Contd...*

*Contd...*

| Substance | Original IDLH value | Revised IDLH value |
|---|---|---|
| Terphenyl (o, m, p isomers) | Unknown | 500 mg/m$^3$ |
| 1,1,1,2-Tetrachloro 2,2-difluoroethane | 15,000 ppm | 2,000 ppm |
| 1,1,2,2-Tetrachloro 1,2-difluoroethane | 15,000 ppm | 2,000 ppm |
| 1,1,2,2-Tetrachloroethane | 150 ppm | 100 ppm |
| Tetrachloroethylene | 500 ppm | 150 ppm |
| Tetrachloronaphthalene | Unknown | Unknown [Unch] |
| Tetraethyl lead (as Pb) | 40 mg Pb/m$^3$ | 40 mg Pb/m$^3$ [Unch] |
| Tetrahydrofuran | 20,000 ppm [LEL] | 2,000 ppm [LEL] |
| Tetramethyl lead (as Pb) | 40 mg Pb/m$^3$ | 40 mg Pb/m$^3$ [Unch] |
| Tetramethyl succinonitrile | 5 ppm | 5 ppm [Unch] |
| Tetranitromethane | 5 ppm | 4 ppm |
| Tetryl | No evidence | 750 mg/m$^3$ |
| Thallium (soluble compounds, as Tl) | 20 mg Tl/m$^3$ | 15 mg Tl/m$^3$ |
| Thiram | 1,500 mg/m$^3$ | 100 mg/m$^3$ |
| Tin (inorganic compounds, as Sn) | 400 mg Sn/m$^3$ | 100 mg Sn/m$^3$ |
| Tin (organic compounds, as Sn) | Unknown | 25 mg Sn/m$^3$ |
| Titanium dioxide | No evidence | 5,000 mg/m$^3$ |
| Toluene | 2,000 ppm | 500 ppm |
| Toluene 2,4-diisocyanate | 10 ppm | 2.5 ppm |
| o-Toluidine | 100 ppm | 50 ppm |
| Tributyl phosphate | 125 ppm | 30 ppm |
| 1,1,2-Trichloroethane | 500 ppm | 100 ppm |
| Trichloroethylene | 1,000 ppm | 1,000 ppm [Unch] |
| Trichloronaphthalene | Unknown | Unknown [Unch] |
| 1,2,3-Trichloropropane | 1,000 ppm | 100 ppm |
| 1,1,2-Trichloro 1,2,2-trifluoroethane | 4,500 ppm | 2,000 ppm |
| Triethylamine | 1,000 ppm | 200 ppm |
| Trifluorobromomethane | 50,000 ppm | 40,000 ppm |
| 2,4,6-Trinitrotoluene | 1,000 mg/m$^3$ | 500 mg/m$^3$ |
| Triorthocresyl phosphate | 40 mg/m$^3$ | 40 mg/m [Unch] |
| Triphenyl phosphate | No evidence | 1,000 mg/m$^3$ |
| Turpentine | 1,500 ppm | 800 ppm |
| Uranium (insoluble compounds, as U) | 30 mg U/m$^3$ | 10 mg U/m$^3$ |
| Uranium (soluble compounds, as U) | 20 mg U/m$^3$ | 10 mg U/m$^3$ |
| Vanadium dust | 70 mg/m (as V2O5) | 35 mg V/m$^3$ |

*Contd...*

*Contd...*

| | | |
|---|---|---|
| Vanadium fume | 70 mg/m (as V2O5) | 35 mg V/m$^3$ |
| Vinyl toluene | 5,000 ppm | 400 ppm |
| Warfarin | 350 mg/m$^3$ | 100 mg/m$^3$ |
| Xylene (o, m, p isomers) | 1,000 ppm | 900 ppm |
| Xylidine | 150 ppm | 50 ppm |
| Yttrium compounds (as Y) | No evidence | 500 mg Y/m$^3$ |
| Zinc chloride fume | 4,800 mg/m$^3$ | 50 mg/m$^3$ |
| Zinc oxide | 2,500 mg/m$^3$ | 500 mg/m$^3$ |
| Zirconium compounds (as Zr) | 500 mg Zr/m$^3$ | 25 mg Zr/m$^3$ |

the UN Recommendations on the Transport of Dangerous Goods, which form the basis for most regional and national regulatory schemes. For instance, the International Civil Aviation Organization has developed regulations for air transport of hazardous materials that are based upon the UN Model but modified to accommodate unique aspects of air transport. Individual airline and governmental requirements are incorporated with this by the International Air Transport Association to produce the widely used IATA Dangerous Goods Regulations (DGR). Similarly, the International Maritime Organization has developed the International Maritime Dangerous Goods Code ("IMDG Code", part of the International Convention for the Safety of Life at Sea) for transportation on the high seas, and the Intergovernmental Organization for International Carriage by Rail has developed the Regulations Concerning the International Carriage of Dangerous Goods by Rail ("RID", part of the Convention Concerning International carriage by Rail). Many individual nations have also structured their dangerous goods transportation regulations to harmonize with the UN Model in organization as well as in specific requirements. The Globally Harmonized System of Classification and Labeling of Chemicals (GHS) is an internationally agreed upon system set to replace the various classification and labeling standards used in different countries. GHS will use consistent criteria for classification and labeling on a global level (Figure 2.2).

## International Regulatory Bodies

| Air | ICAO | International Civil Aviation Organization |
|---|---|---|
| Sea | IMO | International Maritime Organization |
| Road | ADR | International Carriage of Dangerous Goods by Road |
| Rail | RID | International Carriage of Dangerous Goods by Rail |

### *International Civil Aviation Organization – International Air Transport Association*

In practice the IATA Dangerous Goods Regulations (DGR) Manual is the industry standard for transportation of dangerous goods by air. It provides all provisions mandated by International Civil Aviation Organisation (ICAO), and all rules agreed by airlines for safely handling of dangerous goods.

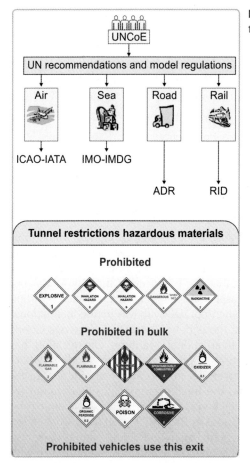

**Figure 2.2** UN recommendations for transport of dangerous chemicals

### International Maritime Organization – International Maritime Dangerous Goods

The principal international rules for the carriage of packaged dangerous goods by sea are published in the International Maritime Dangerous Goods Code (IMDG Code). The IMDG Code is updated and published by the International Maritime Organisation (IMO). The Code is based on the UN Recommendations on the Transport of Dangerous Goods but also includes additional requirements applicable to the transport of hazardous materials by sea (e.g. requirements for marine pollutants, freight containers, stowage and segregation as well other requirements applicable to shipboard safety and preservation of the marine environment) that are not covered by the UN Recommendations.

### International Carriage of Dangerous Goods by Road

European Agreement concerning the International Carriage of Dangerous Goods by Road.

## *International Carriage of Dangerous Goods by Rail*

The International Carriage of Dangerous Goods by Rail within Europe is governed by the Convention Concerning International Carriage by Rail (COTIF).

## DISPOSAL OF CHEMICAL WASTE

Guidelines are different for hazardous and extremely hazardous chemical waste.

### Designate a Hazardous Waste Storage Area

- Select an area that is:
  - Near where the waste is generated
  - Under the control of laboratory personnel
  - Out of the way of normal laboratory activities
- Label the area with a "Danger – Hazardous Waste" sign
- Make the area easily accessible and recognizable to waste technicians
- **Note:** Fume hoods may be used to temporarily store small quantities of waste materials, but should not serve as designated waste storage areas.

### Select Appropriate Containers

- **Chemical compatibility**
  - Choose a container chemically compatible with the material it will hold
  - Chemicals must not react with, weaken, or dissolve the container or lid
  - Follow these basic compatibility guidelines:
    - Acids or bases: Do not store in metal
    - Hydrofluoric acid: Do not store in glass
    - Gasoline (solvents): Do not store or transport in lightweigh polyethylene containers such as milk jugs
- **Caps and closure**
  - Use waste containers with leak-proof, screw-on caps so contents cannot leak if a container tips over. Corks, parafilm, and beakers are not acceptable
  - If necessary, transfer waste material to a container that can be securely closed. Label the new container
  - Keep waste containers closed except when adding waste
  - Wipe down containers prior to your scheduled collection date.
- **Size**
  - Choose appropriately sized containers. Store smaller quantities in smaller containers. It is not cost-effective to dispose of 50 milliliters of material in a 4 liter container.
- **Secondary containment**
  - Always place your container in a secondary container to:
    - Capture spills and leaks from the primary container

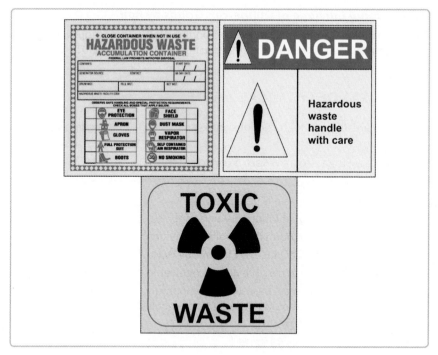

**Figure 2.3** Chemical hazard waste signs

    ♦  Segregate incompatible hazardous wastes, such as acids and bases
- A secondary container must be chemically compatible and able to hold 110% of the volume of waste stored in the primary container(s). Laboratory trays and dish pans are frequently used for secondary containment.
- **Label every waste container with a hazardous waste tag**
  - Attach a completed hazardous waste tag to the container before you begin using the container to accumulate and store waste (Figure 2.3).
  - Cross out all other labels on the container. (Do not obliterate the original product label; waste technicians need to see what the container held before it was designated as a waste receptacle.)
- **Liquid waste requirements**
  - Do not overfill liquid waste containers. Leave a sizable amount of head space in the container to allow for expansion and safe transportation — 10% head space is a good rule of thumb.
  - Do not mix solids with liquid waste. Containers found to contain solids during processing by EH&S hazardous waste technicians will be returned to the generator for separation.
- **Liquid-filled small containers** such as vials and Eppendorf tubes:
  - Double-bag containers in clear plastic bags to allow visual inspection by waste technicians

- Containers bagged together must contain liquids or liquid mixtures with the same chemical constituents
- Seal each bag individually
- Accurately list the bag's contents and chemical constituents on the hazardous waste tag.
- **Organic solvents**
  - Halogenated and non-halogenated organic solvents may be mixed together in the same waste container. Do not combine organic solvents with toxic metal waste!
  - Safety officer should follow the proper regulations and guidelines in the case of using toxic metal compounds include arsenic, barium, cadmium, chromium, lead, mercury, selenium, silver, copper, nickel, and zinc.

### Dry, Solid Waste

Chemically contaminated solid waste includes 3 categories that are packaged differently for disposal: Laboratory trash, dry chemicals, and sharps and piercing objects.

- **Laboratory trash:** Examples include absorbent paper products, wipes, gloves, bench coat, and other laboratory supplies. Follow these guidelines:
  - Double- plastic bags bag the waste in clear to allow visual inspection by waste technicians
  - Seal each bag individually
  - Accurately list the bag's contents and chemical constituents on the hazardous waste tag.
- **Dry chemicals:**
  - Dispose of solid reagent chemicals in the manufacturer's container.
  - Label the container with a hazardous waste tag.
- **Sharps and piercing objects:** Sharps are items capable of puncturing, piercing, or tearing regular waste bags. Examples include pipettes, pipette tips, and broken glass. Sharps require special packaging.

### Empty Containers that Once Held Hazardous Chemicals

Disposal of these containers depends on the container's size, what it is made of, and the hazardous material it once contained.

### Guidelines for "Unknowns" or Unidentified Chemical Waste

Processing and disposal of unknowns is particularly expensive because they must be handled with great care and caution. Please make every effort to avoid "unknowns" by diligently labeling and dating inventory.

- Once found, ask others working in the area if they know what the material is.
- If the material can be identified:
  - Label it with a hazardous waste tag
- If the material cannot be identified:
  - Label it with a hazardous waste tag

- Write "Unknown" on the tag
- Write on the waste tag any known information. Include:
    ◆ Type of laboratory that material was found in (chemistry, organic or inorganic, biology, DNA research, etc.)
    ◆ Where the material was discovered in the laboratory (under a fume hood with other organics, on a shelf with inorganics or salts, etc.)
    ◆ Age of the material.
- Request a hazardous waste collection.

## Storage Time and Quantity Limits Before Waste must be Collected

Request a hazardous waste collection before time or quantity limits are reached.

- Time: All hazardous waste must be collected within 90 days from when waste is first put into containers.
- Quantity: Up to 55 gallons of any individual hazardous waste may be stored before it must be collected.
    - When 55 gallons or more of hazardous waste accumulates, the waste must be collected within 3 days.

# Chapter Three

# Radioactive Materials Hazard

## INTRODUCTION

Radioactive materials can be in the form of open sources or sealed sources. An open source of radioactive material is normally used as a tracer in experiments and has the potential for spillage and release if not properly contained. A sealed source is in a form that is permanently bonded or fixed in a capsule or matrix designed to prevent release of the radioactive material.

### The Major Types of Radiation

- **Alpha particles**—massive charged particles, identical in mass and charge with 4He nuclei that are emitted from the nucleus with discrete energies (for example, 238U alpha particles).
- **Beta particles**—light charged particles that come in positive (positron) and negative (negatron) forms, have the same mass as an electron and are emitted from the nucleus with a continuous range of energies up to some maximum energy (for example, 22Na emits positrons, 32P, 3H, 14C, 35S and 131I all emit negatrons).
- **Gamma rays**—electromagnetic radiation emitted from the nucleus with discrete energies (for example, 131I, 125I, 57Co, 51Cr, 137Cs).
- **X-rays**—electromagnetic radiation emitted from the electron shells of an atom with discrete energies (for example, 131I, 125I).

Two other types of radiation are generated in the material surrounding the radioactive atoms rather than by the radioactive atoms themselves. These are external bremsstrahlung and annihilation radiation.

- **External bremsstrahlung**—consists of photons created by the acceleration of changed particles in the electromagnetic field of the nucleus. The photons are emitted with a continuous range of energies up to the maximum energy of the charged particle. For example, when phosphorous-32 (32P) beta particles interact with certain materials, for example, lead, significant external bremsstrahlung radiation fields can be generated.
- **Annihilation radiation**—consists of two 0.511 MeV photons formed by the mutual annihilation of a positive beta particle and an electron. For example, when sodium-22 (22Na) positive beta particles interact with matter, annihilation radiation is emitted.

## RADIOACTIVE SYMBOL

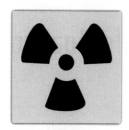

Radioactivity sign.

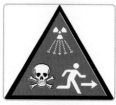

Ionizing radiation (new sign).

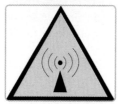

Non-ionizing radiation sign.

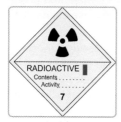

The maximum allowable radioactivity is 0.5 mR/hr on the package surface.

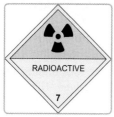

Vehicles carrying packages with yellow labels must have a radioactive placard on both sides and both ends of the vehicle.

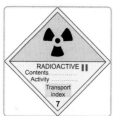

The maximum allowable radioactivity is 50 mR/hr on the package surface, and one mR/hr at three feet from the package.

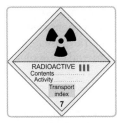

Maximum allowable radioactivity is 200 mR/hr on the package surface, and 10 mR/hr at three feet from the package. Required for fissile Class III materials or large quantity shipments of any radiation level.

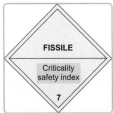

Applied to packages that contain fissile materials.

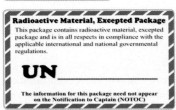

Empty-applied to packages that have been emptied of contents, but may contain regulated amounts of internal contamination and minimal radiation levels detectable outside of the package (less than 0.5 mR/hr).

## RADIATION MEASUREMENTS

**Roentgen:** It is the measurement of energy produced by Gamma or X-Ray radiation in acubic centimeter of air. It is abbreviated with the capital "R". One milliroentgen, abbreviated "mR" is one-thousandth of a roentgen. One microroentgen, abbreviated "uR" is one-millionth of a roentgen.

**RAD:** Radiation Absorbed Dose. Original measuring unit for expressing the absorption of all types of ionizing radiation (alpha, beta, gamma, neutrons, etc) into any medium. One rad is equivalent to the absorption of 100 ergs of energy per gram of absorbing tissue.

**REM:** Roentgen Equivalent Man is a measurement that correlates the dose of any radiation to the biological effect of that radiation. Since not all radiation has the same biological effect, the dosage is multiplied by a "quality factor" (Q). For example, a person receiving a dosage of gamma radiation will suffer much less damage than a person receiving the same dosage from alpha particles, by a factor of three. So alpha particles will cause three times more damage than gamma rays. Therefore, alpha radiation has a quality factor of three. Following is the Q factor for a few radiation types:

| Radiation | Quality factor (Q) |
|---|---|
| Beta, gamma and X-rays | 1 |
| Thermal neutrons | 3 |
| Fast n, a, and protons | 10 |
| Heavy and recoil nuclei | 20 |

The difference between the rad and rem is that the rad is a measurement of the radiation absorbed by the material or tissue. The rem is a measurement of the biological effect of that absorbed radiation. For general purposes, most physicists agree that the Roentgen, Rad and Rem may be considered equivalent.

## System International (SI) of Units

The System International of Unit for radiation measurements is now the official system of measurements. This system uses the "gray" (Gy) and "sivert" (Sv) for absorbed dose and equivalent dose respectively.

## The Conversion from One System to Another is Simple

| | |
|---|---|
| 1 Sv = 100 rem | 1 rem = .01 Sv |
| 1 mSv = 100 mR (mrem) | 1 mR = .01 mSv |
| 1 Gy = 100 rad | 1 rad = .01 Gy |
| 1mGy = 100 mrad | 1 mrad = .01 mGy |

## Radioactive Substances Hazards

The hazards to people and the environment from radioactive contamination depend on the nature of the radioactive contaminant, the level of contamination, and the extent of the spread of contamination. The higher the dose the greater the severity, examples of such proportional effects are erythema (reddening of the skin), epilation (loss of hair), cataracts and "acute radiation syndrome". Serious birth defects, carcinogenesis and radiation mutagenesis which is the induction of changes in hereditary traits caused by radiation damage to the chromosomes.

### Low Level Contamination

Low levels of radioactive contamination pose little risk. In the case of low-level contamination by isotopes with a short half-life, the best course of action may be to simply allow the material to naturally decay. Longer-lived isotopes should be cleaned up and properly disposed of, because even a very low level of radiation can be life-threatening when in long exposure to it. Therefore, whenever there is any radiation in an area, many people take extreme caution when approaching.

### High Level Contamination

High levels of contamination may pose major risks to people and the environment. People can be exposed to potentially lethal radiation levels, both externally and internally, from the spread of contamination following an accident (or a deliberate initiation) involving large quantities of radioactive material. The biological effects of external exposure to radioactive contamination are generally the same as those from an external radiation source not involving radioactive materials, such as X-ray machines, and are dependent on the absorbed dose.

### Biological Effects

The biological effects of internally deposited radionuclides depend greatly on the activity and the bio distribution and removal rates of the radionuclide, which in turn depends on its chemical form. The biological effects may also depend on the chemical toxicity of the deposited material, independent of its radioactivity. Some radionuclides may be generally distributed throughout the body and rapidly removed, as is the case with tritiated water. Some radionuclides may target specific organs and have much lower removal rates. For instance, the thyroid gland takes up a large percentage of any iodine that enters the body. If large quantities of radioactive iodine are inhaled or ingested, the thyroid may be impaired or destroyed, while other tissues are affected to a lesser extent. Radioactive iodine is a common fission product; it was a major component of the radiation released from the Chernobyl disaster, leading to many cases of pediatric thyroid cancer and hypothyroidism. On the other hand, radioactive iodine is used in the diagnosis and treatment of many diseases of the thyroid precisely because of the thyroid's selective uptake of iodine.

## General Safety Precautions

- Warnings sign must be posted in work and storage areas.
- In laboratories that use unsealed radioactive material or other hazardous materials, no eating or drinking is allowed anywhere in the laboratory. No storage of food or beverages for human consumption is allowed in laboratories, cold rooms, freezers, deli coolers or refrigerators used for storage or use of hazardous materials, including radioactive materials.
- Appropriate shielding must be used for gamma, neutron, and high-energy beta emitting radionuclide work: low-density material such as plexiglass or wood for beta emitters, high-density material such as lead for gamma emitters or X-rays, and hydrogenous material (water, paraffin, masonite) for neutron emitters.
- Properly dress and cover open wounds before working with radioactive materials.
- Wear a dosimeter properly and when required.
- Use appropriate shielding for each type of radionuclide. For example, shield 32P with 3/8 inch of plexiglass. 125I can be shielded with 1/8 inch of lead sheeting or lead glass equivalent.
- Use mechanical devices such as tongs, clamps, tweezers, etc. when manipulating radioactive materials to help minimize exposure.
- Handle and store radioactive material only in specifically designated and authorized locations. Posting must include the message:
  Caution—Radioactive material and display the radiation symbol when required. Doors of refrigerators and incubators in which radioactive materials are stored and doors to laboratories using radioactive materials must be labeled.
- Remember, time, distance and shielding are the means of reducing the radiation dose when working with radioactive material. Plan work in advance to save time. Use tongs, clamps, tweezers, etc. to provide distance from the source. Use appropriate shielding to reduce the radiation.
- Use disposable absorbent material with impervious backing to cover work surfaces wherever radioactive material is used. Clearly label the work area with radioactive tape and identify the radionuclide and amount of radioactive material in use.

- When opening or handling volatile radionuclides or those with the potential to volatilize, use radioisotope fume hoods. Unbound 125I or 131I (NaI) can be more volatile at lower pH's. Large amounts of 35S have been known to volatilize. Products labeled with 3H (tritium) can be volatile when stored in a chemical solvent. Tritiated products become especially volatile when the solvent is evaporated.
- Properly survey the work area for contamination during and after each procedure and at the end of the day. If any contamination is found, decontaminate before leaving the work area.
- Store radioactive material in clearly labeled and tightly closed containers. Secure against unauthorized removal. If stock vials are left unattended for more than five minutes, they should be locked up or the room itself should be locked.
- Only dispose of radioactive materials in specially designated and clearly identified waste containers. Do not use biohazard bags for radioactive wastes. Radioactive liquid waste must be completely absorbed before disposal. If liquid scintillation vials are used, EH&S will accept plastic and glass liquid scintillation vials for pickup.
- Sharps contaminated with radioactive material must be placed in sharps containers labeled for radioactive material.

## PERSONAL SAFETY

### Laboratory Coat and Apron

Disposable laboratory coats are best for working around long-lived radionuclides. Reusable laboratory coats are acceptable when handling short-lived radionuclides, provided they are stored for a sufficient time to permit decay of any contamination prior to being washed.

Both cloth and disposable laboratory coats may be reused if they are free from contamination and in good condition. They should be stored in a controlled area and laboratory coats should be monitor both during operations and after removing them. Particular attention should be paid to the sleeves, pockets and lower front surfaces of the coat. All laboratory coats should be fire-resistant. Waterproof aprons, full-body jump suits and hoods provide additional protection in environments where the potential for more severe contamination is present.

### Gloves

Gloves are secondary protection only. They should not be used to handle radioactive materials directly. When no longer need gloves, they should be carefully removed, monitored and disposed or stored appropriately. Rips or holes make gloves ineffective. Periodic changes of gloves are recommended. The greater the potential hazard, the more frequent a change of gloves is needed. Wearing two pair of gloves and frequently changing the outer pair is also a good safety practice. Gloves should be monitored frequently. If gloves are exposed to radionuclides that emit penetrating radiation, it should be removed quickly as possible to minimize skin exposure. This is particularly important when handling high-energy beta emitters.

## Footwear

Comfortable, sturdy footwear should be selected that will protect against contamination. Sandals or open-toe shoes are not allowed. In controlled areas where low-level floor contamination is a potential hazard, a separate pair of work shoes for use only in that area is a good idea. Disposable shoe covers of plastic or paper are available to prevent contamination of ordinary shoes. However, these can wear through rapidly and can be slippery.

## Eye and Face Protection

Safety glasses are of some use in protecting against low penetration radiation, such as low-energy X-rays and medium-energy beta particles but provide little protection from penetrating gamma radiation.

## Respiratory Protection

Contain operations that create radioactive dust, vapor or gases. Vented enclosures with protective filters are available for such operations. In cases where entering a contaminated zone is unavoidable or in emergency situations, respiratory protection may be necessary.

## Personal Monitoring

After each procedure and before leaving the area, monitor hands, shoes, and laboratory coat for contamination using an appropriate radiation detection instrument.

## Radiation Protection Dosimetry

- External dosimetry, where the radiation source is outside the body and the biological properties of the source do not influence the dose equivalent received.

External dosimetry is commonly performed by one or both of the following methods:

- Personal dosimeter, that indicates the dose equivalent at a point on the body.
- The dose equivalent is estimated by considering the dose equivalent rate in the area and how long you worked there. The dose equivalent rate might be measured or calculated.
- Personal dosimeters.

The most common personal dosimeters are a film dosimeter, thermoluminescent dosimeter (TLD), optically stimulated luminescent dosimeters (OSLD) and pocket ionization chamber (PIC or "pencil dosimeter"). Film dosimeters consist of a small piece of photographic film in a light-proof package. Filters are placed over the film to obtain information about the type and energy of the incident radiation. This information is needed to adjust the dose equivalent indicated by the film because the film does not respond to radiation in exactly the same way as tissue. Film dosimeters fade and are sensitive to heat. They have the advantages of being relatively inexpensive and providing a permanent record of the dose equivalent received.

TLDs are small inorganic crystals that, when heated, emit a quantity of light. Under certain conditions, the light emitted is proportional to the energy deposited in the crystal. TLDs are small, rugged, reusable and respond to most types of radiation in the same way as tissue. However, TLDs are more expensive than film dosimeters and do not provide a permanent record of the dose equivalent.

OSLDs are similar to TLDs except that the absorbed radiation energy is released by laser light instead of heat. These dosimeters are also small and rugged, can be reanalyzed and are more sensitive than TLDs.

PICs are small ionization chambers that are relatively expensive and not very rugged. Direct reading PICs may be read in the field without erasing the accumulated dose. This provides an immediate reading of the dose equivalent being received during an operation, which is very helpful in reducing doses.

Personal dosimeters should be worn on the part of your body that receives the greatest dose in relation to its dose limit. Preferably, several dosimeters should be worn at key locations. Dosimeters should be stored in an area where there is a low, constant background. They should be kept free of contamination.

• Estimating dose equivalents

The dose equivalent you receive can be estimated by measuring the dose rate with a survey meter and multiplying by the length of time you stay in the radiation field. This method is useful for estimating the magnitude of the dose likely to be received. However, problems can arise when the dose equivalent rate is incorrectly measured, the dose equivalent rate measured is not representative of the radiation fields where you work or the time you will spend in the field is underestimated.

• Internal dosimetry, where the radiation source is inside the body and the dose equivalent received depends on the biological properties of the source.

The distribution and retention of a radioactive material will influence the dose equivalent received once it is inside the body. Therefore, in internal dosimetry, you do not try to directly measure dose; instead, you characterize the distribution and retention of the radioactive material. Once this is known, the dose equivalent can be readily calculated using standard internal dosimetry methods.

## RADIOACTIVE MATERIAL STORAGE

• All radioactive materials must be secured from unauthorized use or removal at all times; secure stock solutions of radioactive material or sealed/plated sources in a locked storage area and/or laboratory room when left unattended.

• Stock solutions of radioactive materials, sealed/plated sources, and radioactive wastes must never be stored in an unrestricted and non-posted area or facility.

• Designated radionuclide work and storage areas must be clearly identified and all equipment or containers used for radionuclide work must be labeled properly with radioactive material warning tape.

• Refrigerators and freezers used to store radionuclides must be clearly labeled with specific labels.

## Radiation Spill Response

Spreading of radiation beyond the spill area can easily occur by the movement of personnel involved in the spill or cleanup effort.

### Minor Radiation Spill

1. Alert people in the immediate area of the spill.
2. Wear protective equipment, including safety goggles, disposable gloves, shoe covers, and long-sleeve laboratory coat.
3. Place absorbent paper towels over liquid spill. Place towels dampened with water or decontaminant cleaner over spills of solid materials.
4. Using forceps or gloved hand, placed towels in plastic bag. Dispose in radiation waste container.
5. Monitor area, hands, and shoes for contamination with an appropriate survey meter. Repeat cleanup until contamination is no longer detected.

### Major Radiation Spill

1. Attend to injured or contaminated persons and remove them from exposure.
2. Alert people in the laboratory to evacuate.
3. Have potentially contaminated personnel stay in one area until they have been monitored and shown to be free of contamination.
4. Call the Radiation Safety Officer and Radiation Safety Personnel.
5. Close the doors and prevent entrance into affected area.

## Radioactive Material Waste Processing

1. Use clear or black plastic bags for collection only. This includes smaller bags used for bench top waste. Waste must be dry with no moisture visible inside the bags.
2. Fill out waste form completely before turning it into radiation safety for waste pick up.
3. Separate solid waste by half-life. A short half-life is less than to 300 days. Long half-life is greater than 300 days.
4. For bulk liquid wastes use sturdy plastic containers. Lids to all containers must be sealed completely to prevent leakage during transport. If liquid waste is water soluble then all isotopes can be placed together in the container.
5. If the liquid waste is not water soluble put this waste in a separate container and identify the contents.
6. Packages containing radioactive material should be labeled knowing the level of radiation contained.
   - A white Level I label means there is such a low level of radiation that you face very little to no health risks.
   - A yellow Level II level means there may be some radiation outside the containment package.
   - A yellow Level III label, or a label labeled "FISSILE," contains the highest amount of radiation threat.
7. Avoid storing packages of radioactive material together, as this increases the total net amount of radiation that may come in contact with. Never group more than fifty packages of radioactive material together, and keep

groups of radioactive material six meters from other groups of radioactive material.

8. Implement precautionary safety measures in case a box or package containing radioactive material is broken or opened accidentally. Never touch an opened package and alert others to stay away.

## Liquid Scintillation Vials and Cocktail Waste

1. Separate and pack vials containing only P-32 and/or S-35 in scintillation fluid from other liquid scintillation vials.
2. Place all radioactive liquid scintillation vials in the original trays in the upright position.
   a. Return trays, in the upright position, to the original shipping boxes.
   b. Tape box closed and clearly mark the "up" direction on the outside of the box.
3. If the original container is not available or vials were bought in bulk:
   a. Choose a sturdy cardboard box or metal can of a size, which will accommodate no more than 500 standard vials or 1,000 sub-mini vials.
   b. Line the container with a plastic bag and then place a layer of absorbent paper in the bag.
   c. Place another plastic bag on top of the absorbent paper. This is where the vials will be placed.
   d. Seal both plastic bags when full.
4. If the scintillation vials contain (H-3, C-14, or I-125) and the fluid is less than or equal to 0.05 uCi, then place the scintillation fluid in a container (Please mark this container stating that it contains scintillation fluid) and dispose of the vials in the regular trash.
5. If the scintillation vials containing (H-3, C-14, or I-125) and the fluid is greater than 0.05 uCi, then follow steps 2 and 3, and label the container and/or the bags as high concentration.

## Packaging

All shipments of radioactive materials whether form industry or government, must be packaged and transported according to strict regulations. These regulations protect the public, transportation workers, and the environment from potential exposure to radiation.

### Types of Packaging

The most effective way to reduce the risk associated with transporting radioactive materials is to follow the appropriate packaging standards specified by DOT and, when required, NRC or DOE regulations. The type of packaging used is determined by the activity, type, and form of the material to be shipped. Depending on these factors, radioactive material is shipped in one of three types of containers.

1. Industrial packaging: Materials that present little hazard from radiation exposure, due to their low level of radioactivity, are shipped in industrial packages. These are also known as strong, tight containers. This type of container will retain and protect the contents during normal transportation activities.

2. Type A packages: Radioactive materials with higher specific activity levels, these packages must demonstrate their ability to withstand a series of tests without releasing the contents. Regulations require that the package protect its contents and maintain sufficient shielding under conditions normally encountered during transportation.

3. Type B packages: Radioactive materials that exceed the limits of Type A package requirements must be shipped in Type B packages. Shippers use this type of package to transport materials that would present a radiation hazard to the public or the environment.

## Labels

Labels identify the contents and radioactivity level according to three categories:

1. Radioactive white I: Almost no radiation. The maximum allowable radioactivity is 0.5 mR/hr on the package surface.

2. Radioactive yellow II: Low radiation levels. The maximum allowable radioactivity is 50 mR/hr on the package surface, and one mR/hr at three feet from the package.

3. Radioactive yellow III: Higher levels of radiation. Maximum allowable radioactivity is 200 mR/hr on the package surface, and 10 mR/hr at three feet from the package.

The Yellow II and Yellow III labels have additional items called the transport index box. (The top of the diamonds for 3 Radioactive II and III are actually yellow.) For the majority of shipments, the number in the transport index box indicates the maximum radiation level measured (in mR/hr) at one meter from the surface of the package.

In the examples above, a transport index of 0.1 on the Radioactive III label indicates that radiation measured 1 meter from the surface of the package should be less than 0.1 mR/hr. With the exception of exclusive use shipments, the maximum transport index for any shipment is 10 mR/hr. Packages that carry radioactive materials are designed to absorb radiation if it is released from the container.

## ▌TRANSPORTATION

### Types of Shipments

Radioactive materials that are shipped include:

- Radioisotopes are transported from reactors to medical facilities, research laboratories and defense sites, as well as to a variety of industries and manufacturing facilities.
- Radioactive waste results from processes that use radioactive materials and must be transported to storage or disposal sites (Table 3.1 shipping names as approved by UN).

### Route of Transportation

- Transportation by highway: Trucks transport a wide variety of both low-level and high-level radioactive materials, including fission products used to manufacture nuclear fuel. Transportation of these materials is highly regulated.

■ **Table 3.1** UN numbers and proper shipping names

| UN Number | UN proper shipping name |
| --- | --- |
| 2908 | Radioactive material, excepted package, empty packaging |
| 2909 | Radioactive material, excepted package, articles manufactured from depleted uranium or natural uranium or natural thorium |
| 2910 | Radioactive material, excepted package, limited quantity of material |
| 2911 | Radioactive material, excepted package, instruments or articles |
| 2912 | Radioactive material, low specific activity (LSA-I) non-fissile or fissile excepted |
| 2913 | Radioactive material, surface contaminated objects (SCO-I or SCO-II) non-fissile or fissile excepted |
| 2915 | Radioactive material, type A package, non-fissile or fissile excepted |
| 2916 | Radioactive material, type B(U) package, non-fissile or fissile excepted |
| 2917 | Radioactive material, type B(M) package, non-fissile or fissile excepted |
| 3321 | Radioactive material, low specific activity material (LSA-II), non-fissile or fissile excepted |
| 3322 | Radioactive material, low specific activity material (LSA-III), non-fissile or fissile excepted |
| 3323 | Radioactive material, type C package, non-fissile or fissile excepted |
| 3324 | Radioactive material, low specific activity (LSA-II), fissile |
| 3325 | Radioactive material, low specific activity (LSA-III), fissile |
| 3326 | Radioactive material, surface contaminated objects (SCO-I or SCO-II), fissile |
| 3327 | Radioactive material, type A package, fissile non-special form |
| 3328 | Radioactive material, type B(U) package, fissile |
| 3329 | Radioactive material, type B(M) package, fissile |
| 3330 | Radioactive material, type C package, fissile |
| 3332 | Radioactive material, type A package, special form, non-fissile or fissile excepted |
| 3333 | Radioactive material, type A package, special form, fissile |

- Transportation by Rail: This is the second most frequent method of transporting radioactive materials. Generally, trains carry only large volumes of material, The preferred method of shipping radioactive materials and waste is by unit train, which runs directly between its point of origin and its destination.
- Transportation by Air: It is strictly limits air shipment of radioactive materials. One exception is radiopharmaceuticals. Radiopharmaceuticals are radioactive drugs use to diagnose or treat illnesses, and are frequently short-lived, small and light weight. Often they must be delivered quickly to hospitals and medical laboratories, so air shipment is generally the best method. Air transport of radioactive materials is regulated and issued by the International Atomic Energy Agency (IAEA).

- Transportation by Sea: Only a small percentage of radioactive materials are shipped by sea, primarily because this type of transportation is slow and geographically limited. Materials that are occasionally transported via waterways include spent nuclear fuel, uranium metal, uranium hexafluoride, and low-level waste. When shipped by sea, these materials are identified as "marine pollutants" and noted as such on the manifest.

# Chapter Four

# Biosafety—Healthcare-associated Infections and Biocides

## MICROORGANISMS

Microorganisms are very small organisms. They are invisible to the normal human eye. They can only be seen with the help of a microscope. Not all microorganisms are harmful. They are mainly divided into following groups:

- Bacteria
- Fungi
- Virus
- Protozoa.

### Pathogens

Pathogens are disease causing microorganisms present in the environment around us.

### Right Biocide

A biocide with following properties is the right biocide:

- Broad Spectrum antimicrobial activity
- Resistance-free
- Non-corrosive
- User and eco-friendly
- Long-lasting residual activity
- Not neutralized by organic matter, soap, hard water, plastic, etc.
- Aggressive against tough biofilms.

## DISINFECTION

Reducing pathogens or disease causing microorganisms from the environment surrounding us, is known as disinfection. Disinfection is important to prevent - disease occurrence, contamination in medicine and microbiological laboratories and food spoilage. Disinfectants can be divided into three categories:

- **High level**—Kills all organisms except large number of bacterial spores. Mostly alkylating agents. For example; aldehydes, ethylene oxide, ozone, etc.

- **Intermediate level**—Kills most bacteria (including mycobacteria) and viruses. For example; phenols, halogens (chlorine releasing compounds), etc.
- **Low level disinfection**—Kills only some bacteria and viruses. For example; alcohols, heavy metals, etc.

## STERILIZATION

Complete elimination or destruction of all forms of microbial life including spores from any surface/object is known as sterilization.

Spores are resistant, dormant structure formed inside some bacteria (e.g. Bacillus) can survive adverse condition such as heat, desiccation, radiation and chemicals (Figure 4.1). Since they are formed inside the bacterial cells they are also called endospores.

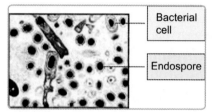

**Figure 4.1** Light microscopic view: A stained preparation of bacteria showing endospores as dark spots and vegetative cells as red

## BIOCIDES

Biocides are chemical agents that kill/inhibit the growth of microorganisms. Biocides are divided into two types.

### Disinfectants

Chemical agents that kill/inhibit the growth of microorganisms (including spores) on non-living/inanimate surfaces.

### Antiseptics

Chemical agents that kill/inhibit the growth of microorganisms (including spores) present on the external surface of the body.

Most chemicals can be used as both depending on the concentration at which they are used. For example, when 5% $H_2O_2$ solution is used for cleaning wounds it acts as an antiseptics and when 10% – 30% $H_2O_2$ is used for bleaching and cleaning non-living surfaces it acts as a disinfectant.

## BIOFILM

A structured community of microorganisms encapsulated within a self-developed polymeric matrix and adherent to a living or inert surface is known

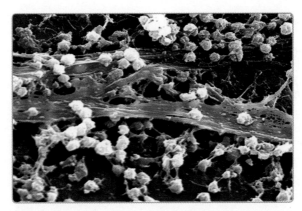

**Figure 4.2** Ultrastructure of biofils forrmed by *Staphylococcus aureus*

as biofilm. Organisms living in a biofilm usually have significantly different properties from free-floating organisms of the same species, as the dense and protected environment of the film allows them to cooperate and interact in various ways. They have increased resistance to biocides and antibiotics as the dense extracellular matrix and the outer layer of cells protect the interior of the community. Biofilms are common in nature, as bacteria have mechanisms by which they can adhere not only to surfaces but to each other too. Biofilms may form on living or non-living surfaces. It represents a prevalent mode of microbial life in natural, industrial and hospital settings. Biofilms can develop on the interiors of pipes and lead to clogging and corrosion biofilms spreading along implanted tubes or wires can lead to pernicious infections in patients. Dental plaque is also a biofilm. Biofilms on floors and counters can make sanitation difficult in food processing/preparation areas (Figure 4.2).

Biofilm development takes place in 5 steps:

1. Initial reversible attachment
2. Irreversible attachment
3. Growth and division of bacteria
4. Exopolymer production and attachment of other organisms
5. Dispersion (Figure 4.3).

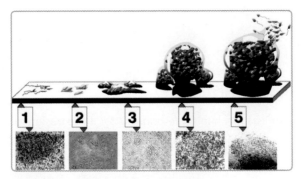

**Figure 4.3** Five steps of biofilm development

## PRIONS

Prions are transmissible (capable of being transmitted) particles, devoid of nucleic acid and seem to be composed exclusively of a modified or misfolded protein (PrPSc), which invariably cause fatal neurodegenerative (a condition in which cells of the brain and spinal cord are lost) diseases. Prion diseases are genetic, infectious, or sporadic disorders, all of which involve modification of the prion protein (PrP). For example, Bovine spongiform encephalopathy (BSE), scrapie of sheep, Creutzfeldt-Jakob disease (CJD).

## DRUG / BIOCIDE RESISTANCE

Drug/biocide resistance is the reduction in effectiveness of a drug/biocide meant to kill the pathogens. Pathogens able to withstand the effect of a drug/biocide are known as drug/biocide resistant pathogens. Pathogens able to withstand the effect of more than one drug/biocide are known as multidrug/biocide resistant pathogens.

Drug/biocide resistance occurs gradually due to:

- Exposure to same drug/biocide over several decades
- Exposed to suboptimal and sublethal levels of drug/biocide
- Extrusion (efflux) of the drug/biocide from the cell.

**Decreasing order of resistance of microorganisms to disinfection and sterilization and the level of disinfection or sterilization.**

| Resistant | Level of disinfection |
|---|---|
| Prions (Creutzfeldt-Jakob disease) | Prion reprocessing |
| Bacterial spores (*Bacillus atrophaeus*) | Sterilization |
| Coccidia (*Cryptosporidium*) | |
| Mycobacteria (*Mycobacterium tuberculosis, Mycobacterium. terrae*) | High |
| Nonlipid or small viruses (polio, coxsackie) | Intermediate |
| Fungi (*Aspergillus, Candida*) | |
| Vegetative bacteria (*Staphylococcus. aureus, Pseudomonas. aeruginosa*) | Low |
| Lipid or medium-sized viruses (HIV, herpes, hepatitis B) | |

**Susceptible**                                    *Modified from Russell and Favero*

## EFFLUX MECHANISM

Efflux mechanism is a mechanism responsible for the extrusion (pushing out) of unwanted toxic substances /antibiotics / biocides, outside the bacterial cell with the help of efflux pumps. Efflux mechanism is an energy dependent mechanism. It contributes to development of bacterial resistance towards antibiotics / biocides (Figure 4.4).

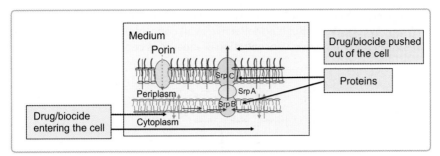

**Figure 4.4** Efflux mechanism

Efflux pump is proteinaceous in nature, located between the two membranes of the bacteria. Some proteins are located within each membrane as well, keeping the structure of the pump and allowing exportation from the inside to the outside of the cell. Mainly drug specific but some may accommodate multiple drugs, causing multidrug resistance.

Efflux pump pushes lot of materials out of the cell using basic protein shape conformations. One protein acts as the docking station, where the drug/biocide fits into the binding pocket. These pockets are normally hydrophobic, so most drugs (excluding large and/or very polar molecules) fit in well. After the molecule is bound to the binding pocket, this protein changes shape, causing the shape change in other proteins, and the molecule is pushed out of the cell. The shapes of the polypeptide chains change depending on the stage they are in. These changes in conformation push the drug out.

## TYPES OF BIOCIDES

Many different types of biocides (antimicrobial agents) are now available that are used for disinfection/antisepsis. They are mainly divided into following groups:

   I.  Alcohols
  II.  Aldehydes
 III.  Biguanides
 IV.  Bisphenols
  V.  Phenols
 VI.  Halogens
VII.  Heavy metals
VIII.  Peroxygens
 IX.  Quaternary ammonium compounds.

### I. Alcohols

Several alcohols possess antimicrobial properties. Alcohols mainly used as biocides are ethanol, methanol and isopropanol. The antimicrobial activity of alcohols can be attributed to their ability to denature proteins. Alcohol solutions containing 60%–95% alcohols are most effective. Concentrations higher than this are less potent as proteins are not denatured easily in the absence of water.

**Ethanol or ethyl alcohol** is rapidly lethal to non-sporulating bacteria and destroys mycobacteria. But it is ineffective at all concentrations against bacterial spores. The most effective concentration of ethanol is between 60–70 %.

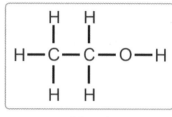

**Ethanol**

**Methanol or methyl alcohol** has poor antimicrobial activity and is not sporicidal. Methanol is potentially toxic too thus, is used rarely.

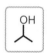

**Methanol**

**Isopropanol/isopropyl alcohol/propan-2-ol/2-propanol** is an isomer of propanol. It is more effective than ethanol but is not sporicidal. Effective concentration of isopropanol is between 60%–70%.

**Mode of action**—alcohols target the proteins present in the cytoplasm and the cytoplasmic membrane. They denature the proteins, cause enzyme inhibition, membrane damage and coagulation of cytoplasmic proteins. These ultimately lead to cell death.

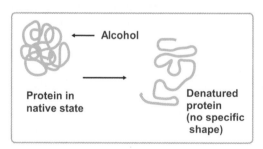

**Mode of action of alcohol**

## II. Aldehydes

There are mainly three aldehydes which are used as disinfectants—formaldehyde, glutaraldehyde and orthophthalaldehyde. Aldehydes possess broad spectrum antimicrobial activity including spores.

**Formaldehyde** is the simplest aldehyde. It is used both as liquid or vapor disinfectant. It kills most bacteria and fungi (including their spores). Formaldehyde is known to be toxic, allergenic, and carcinogenic to humans.

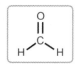

**Formaldehyde**

**Glutaraldehyde is** a dialdehyde colorless liquid with a pungent odor. It is toxic to humans and causes severe eye, nose, throat and lung infection along with headache drowsiness and dizziness. It is a main source of occupational asthma among health care providers.

**Glutaraldehyde**

**Orthophthalaldehyde** abbreviated as OPA, is a dialdehyde. Orthophthalaldehyde is commonly used as a high-level disinfectant for medical instruments.

**Orthophthalaldehyde**

**Mode of action**—aldehydes, target the cell wall, cytoplasmic membrane, cytoplasm and nucleic acids. Aldehydes cross-link with proteins present in the cell wall, react with the thiol, amino, sulfhydryl groups present in the cytoplasm causing protein denaturation and general coagulation of cytoplasm, inhibits normal enzymatic activity and survival functions.

Poly (glutaraldehyde)

$(n + 1)$ PROTEIN—NH$_2$ + Any protein amino group

Cross-linked protein molecules

+ $(n + 1)$ H$_2$O

**Mode of action of aldehydes**

## III. Biguanides

Various biguanides show antimicrobial activity. Biguanides include both mono and polymeric forms. Chlorhexidine and polyhexamethylene biguanide (PHMB) are examples of monomeric and polymeric biguanides respectively.

**Chlorhexidine** is available as a dihydrochloride, diacetate and gluconate. Chlorhexidine has a wide spectrum of antibacterial activity against both Gram-positive and Gram-negative bacteria. It is also tuberculocidal in ethanolic solutions and sporicidal at 98–100°C. The antimicrobial activity of chlorhexidine is only minimally affected by the presence of organic material. It has substantial residual activity. Addition of low concentrations (0.5%–1.0%) of chlorhexidine to alcohol based preparations result in greater residual activity.

**Mode of action**—chlorhexidine targets the lipids present in the cell membrane. It binds to the phosphate and fatty acids of the phospholipids causing membrane damage and leakage of cell components. At high concentrations chlorhexidine causes cytoplasmic coagulation in the bacterial cell.

**Chlorhexidine**

**Polyhexamethylene biguanide (PHMB)** is a disinfectant and a preservative used for skin antisepsis and in surface cleaning solutions. It has very low toxicity to higher organisms such as human cells, which have more complex and protective membranes. PHMB is not cytotoxic and can be directly applied on the skin or wounds.

**Polyhexamethylene biguanide (PHMB)**

**Mode of action**—it has a unique method of action, the polymer strands are incorporated into the bacterial cell wall, which disrupts the membrane and reduces its permeability, and this has a lethal effect on bacteria. It is also known to bind to bacterial DNA, alter its transcription and cause lethal DNA damage.

## IV. Phenols

Phenols also known as phenolics are a class of compounds consisting a hydroxyl group ($OH^-$) bonded to an aromatic hydrocarbon group. The simplest of the class is phenol ($C_6H_5OH$). Some phenols are germicidal and are used in formulating disinfectants.

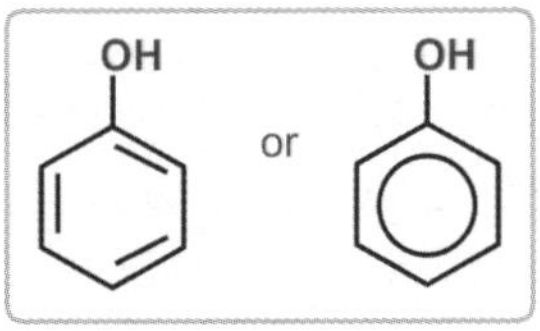

Phenol

**Phenol** is the simplest of the phenols. It is also known as carbolic acid. Phenol has aseptic properties. It was used first time by Joseph Lister for antiseptic surgery. Repeated or prolonged skin contact with phenol may cause dermatitis, and it is a suspected carcinogen. Phenol vapor is corrosive to the eyes, skin and respiratory tract. Also inhalation may cause lung edema. It has harmful effects on the central nervous system, heart and kidneys, resulting in convulsions, coma, cardiac disorders or respiratory failure.

**Chloroxylenol** is used in antimicrobial soaps (Dettol), agar patch studies and isolation of *pseudomonas sp.* It is not significantly toxic to humans and other mammals. It is a mild skin irritant, not sporicidal and has little activity against *Mycobacterium sp.* Chloroxylenol is also inactivated in the presence of organic matter.

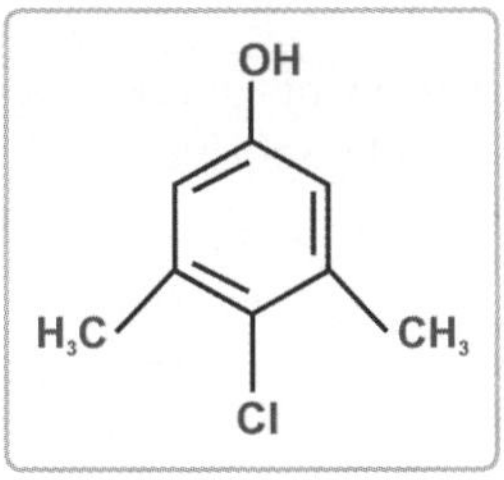

Chloroxylenol

**Mode of action**—the free hydroxyl group is determined to be the reactive components of the phenol molecule. It targets the cell wall and the cytoplasmic membrane of the microorganisms. The initial reaction between a phenolic derivative and bacteria involves binding of the active phenol species to the cell surface. Once the active phenol binds to the exterior of the cell, it penetrates the cell wall either by passive diffusion (Gram-positive) or by the hydrophobic lipid bilayer pathway (Gram-negative). One of the initial events that occur at the cytoplasmic membrane is the inhibition of membrane bound enzymes. Next it damages the cytoplasmic membrane causing the loss in the membrane's ability to act as a permeability barrier leading to leakage of cytoplasmic components and cell death.

## V. Bisphenols

Bisphenols have two phenol functional groups. Bisphenols have potent antibacterial and antifungal activity but have low activity against *Pseudomonas aeruginosa*. Bisphenols have low water solubility.

**Triclosan** is commonly found in a wide range of personal care products such as toothpaste, mouthwash, handwash, soaps, shower foams, deodorants, etc. Its activity is not compromised by organic matter.

**Mode of action**—Triclosan targets the cytoplasmic membrane of the bacterial cell. It also inhibits the fatty acid synthesis necessary for rebuilding cell membrane and reproducing.

## VI. Halogens

Halogens comprise of iodine compounds, chlorine compounds, fluorine and bromine. They are harmful or lethal to organisms.

### *Iodine Compounds*

**Free iodine**—Iodine was first used in the treatment of wounds some 140 years ago. It is an efficient microbicidal agent with rapid lethal activity against bacteria, their spores, fungi and viruses but Iodine efficacy is greatly reduced in the presence of organic matter. It is normally used in aqueous or alcoholic solution. Iodine is less reactive than chlorine.

**Iodophores**—certain surface-active agents can solubilize iodine to form compounds, such as Iodophores (povidone iodine) that retain the biocidal action but not the undesirable properties of iodine. Different concentrations of iodophores are used for antiseptic and disinfectant purposes. Lower concentrations of iodophores used in antisepsis are not sporicidal.

**Chlorine compounds** are commonly used as sanitizing agents in the food industry but are highly irritant and corrosive.

**Hypochlorites** have a wide antibacterial spectrum but are less active against spores and mycobacteria. Two factors that affect the biocidal activity of hypochlorites are organic matter and pH. The hypochlorites are more active at acidic pH than at alkaline pH.

**Sodium hypochlorite** is normally used for the disinfection of swimming pool water.

**Chlorine dioxide** is an alternative to sodium hypochlorite. It retains its biocidal activity over a wide pH range and in the presence of organic matter.

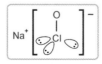
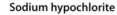
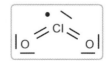

**Sodium hypochlorite**          **Chlorine dioxide**

**Fluorine** is far too toxic, irritant and corrosive to be used as a disinfectant.

**Bromine** is used as disinfectants for drinking water, swimming pools, fresh wounds, spas, dishes, and surfaces.

**Mode of action**—Halogens target cell wall, cytoplasmic membrane and nucleic acids of the bacterial cell. They interfere with the cellular metabolism causing enzyme and nuclear material denaturation, inhibit protein synthesis and loss of integrity in the cell membrane. Halogens also cause lipid and fatty acid degradation causing cell wall damage. They interact with the amino (–NH) and thiol (–SH) groups present in the cytoplasm causing rapid partitioning and disintegration of the cytoplasm.

## VII. Heavy Metals

Heavy metals especially copper, silver and mercury are used as antimicrobial agents. In addition to processing antimicrobial activity these metal ions also help in the activity of other drugs.

**Copper compounds (sulfate, acetate and citrate)** are mainly used as ingredients of antiseptic astringent lotions, in algicides and fungicides.

**Silver compounds Silver** and its compounds (nitrate and sulfadiazine) are known to have antimicrobial properties for thousands of years when silver containers were used to store water for preservation. Silver compounds are used in medicine, prevention of infection in burns, water disinfection, etc.

Silver nitrate          Silver sulfadiazine

**Mercury compounds**—use of mercury has decreased in medicine but a number of organic derivatives of mercury (mercurochrome, nitromersol, thiomersal, phenylmercuric nitrate) are still used as bacteriostatic and fungistatic agents and as bactericides.

**Mode of action**—heavy metals target the cytoplasmic membrane, cytoplasm and nucleic acid of the bacterial cell. These material interact with thiol or sulphydryl (–SH) groups, binds to key functional groups of enzymes and proteins, causes release of potassium ions, inhibit bacterial growth and cell division, causes structural damage to the membrane and ultimately cell death.

## VIII. Peroxygens

**Peroxygens** include hydrogen peroxide, peracetic acid, chlorine dioxide and ozone. This group of biocides are widely used for cleaning, antisepsis, disinfection and sterilization applications. Applications include the use of these biocides in various liquid and gaseous forms, for food and water disinfection and low temperature surface sterilization.

Hydrogen peroxide        Peracetic acid

**Mode of action**—peroxygens target the cell wall, cytoplasmic membrane and cytoplasm.

They interact with the cell surface and break down into $H_2O$ and free $OH^-$ radicals. Free $OH^-$ radicals oxidize all macromolecules such as carbohydrates, lipids, proteins, amino acids and nucleic acid. It also targets the thiol groups in cysteine residues (important determinants of protein structure and function) present in many proteins and vital microbial enzymes. Oxidation of the thiol group results in metabolic inhibition of the cell. Structural proteins in the cell wall, membrane, and ribosomes may also be affected by disruption of stabilizing disulfide cross links between cysteine residues causing disruption of cell membrane, inactivation of enzymes and metabolic inhibition leading to cell death.

**Mode of action of peroxygens**

## IX. Quaternary Ammonium Compounds

Quaternary ammonium compounds (QACs) also known as 'quats' are used as disinfectants, surfactants, fabric softeners and as antistatic agents (e.g. in shampoos). Cetrimide, benzalkonium chloride, didecyl dimethyl ammonium chloride are quats which are used as effective antimicrobial and disinfectants. Other than bacteria quats have good antifungal, antiprotozonic, and antiviral (enveloped) activity. Quats kill just about everything except endospores, *Mycobacterium tuberculosis*, lipid-containing viruses, and *Pseudomonas sp.* (some *Pseudomonas sp.* can even grow in solutions of quats, e.g. cetrimide). Quats are not very effective in the presence of organic compounds.

**Benzalkonium chloride (BKC)** is a nitrogenous cationic surface acting agent. It is a rapidly acting biocidal agent with a moderate residual action. BKC being the first generation quat has lowest relative antimicrobial activity.

**Cetrimide** is first generation quat. It is used as selective media for the growth of *Pseudomonas aeruginosa*. Widely used in the examination of cosmetics, pharmaceuticals and clinical specimens to test for the presence of *P. aeruginosa*.

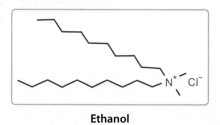

**Didecyl dimethyl ammonium chloride (DDAC)** is the fourth generation (twin or dual chain) quat. It has stronger/superior antimicrobial activity. DDAC has increased tolerance to hard water and organic matter and is low foaming.

**Ethanol**

**Mode of action**—Quats target the cytoplasmic membrane and proteins. They cause disruption of intermolecular interactions, dissociation of lipid bilayers which increases permeability of cell membrane and leakage of cytoplasmic contents. Quats also cause deactivation of enzymes responsible for respiration and metabolic cellular activities, inactivation of energy producing enzymes and denaturation of essential cell proteins, leading to cell death.

## SITES OF ACTION OF DIFFERENT BIOCIDES

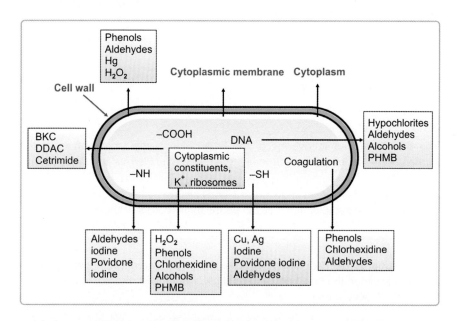

## SITES OF ACTION OF BIOSHIELDS PRODUCTS

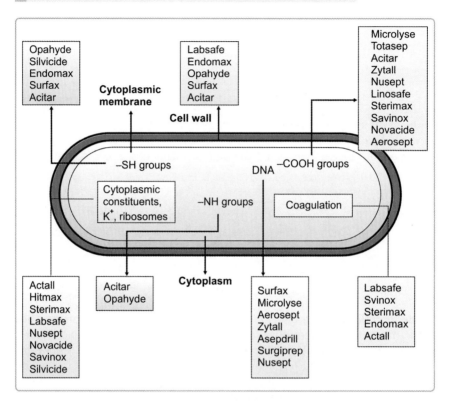

## BIOSAFETY PRODUCTS OF BIOSHIELDS FOR HOSPITALS AND LABORATORIES

There are three main areas of disinfection. They are:

- Skin disinfection
- Environment and surface disinfection
- Laboratory glassware
- Instrument disinfection.

### Skin

The skin is the outer covering of the body. Skin is the largest organ of the human body made up of multiple layers—Epidermis, Dermis and Hypodermis/ Subcutaneous.

Skin plays a key role in protecting the body against pathogens, abrasive actions and excessive water loss. It acts as the permeability barrier to the environment.

### Infection

An infection is defined as the process by which germs/pathogens enter a susceptible site in the host body and multiply, resulting in disease. Infections can be mainly divided into:

## Community Acquired Infections

Infections that are present or incubating at the time of admission to the health care facility and have no association with previous history of hospitalization are known as community acquired infections. For example, Malaria, TB, leprosy, typhoid, measles, dengue.

## Hospital Acquired Infections (HAI) or Nosocomial Infections

Any infection which was absent at the time of admission in the hospital or patient may develop up to 15 days after discharge from the hospital or is acquired by the health care worker during any health care procedure is called hospital acquired /nosocomial infection.

### Surgical Site Infections (SSI)

Surgical site infections are those which occur after the surgery in the part of the body where the surgery took place. SSI include most common nosocomial infections (38%), incisional (2/3rd), organs (1/3rd) and other organs and spaces manipulated during an operation.

## Skin Needs to be Disinfected

The human skin is a rich environment for microbes. Around 1000 species of bacteria are found on the skin. Microflora present on the skin is divided into two groups—transient flora and resident flora.

## Transient Flora

Those bacteria which colonizes the superficial layer, are easier to remove by routine handwash, are most frequently associated with HAI (hospital acquired infections) are known as the transient flora. For example, *Staphylococcus aureus, Pseudomonas sp.*

## Resident Flora

Those bacteria which are attached to deeper layers of the skin and are more resistant to removal are classified as resident flora. For example, CNS (Coagulase-negative staphylococci), Klebsiella, Corynebacteria.

Any break in the skin is a potential site of infection due to the presence of various microorganisms on the skin. For example; surgical site, or site where the IV-catheter, or intravenous catheter is inserted is susceptible to infection. Hence, the skin needs to be disinfected.

### Transmission of Pathogens

Hands are mainly responsible for transmission of pathogens. Hands get contaminated while (Figure 4.5):
- Pulling up patients in the bed
- Checking blood pressure or pulse
- Touching a patients hand
- Rolling patients over in bed
- Touching the patients gown or bedsheets

- Touching equipments like bedside rails, over bed tables, IV pumps
- By touching environmental surfaces near affected patients.

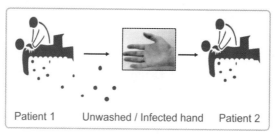

Patient 1      Unwashed / Infected hand      Patient 2

**Figure 4.5** Cross-transmission of pathogens through unwashed hands between patients

## PHLEBOTOMY

It demands the use of SAFE and EFFECTIVE antiseptics that not only have an immediate disinfectant effect, but also good residual activity to protect the patient not only during but also after phlebotomy. The use of uncharacterized dubious alcohols / methylated spirits have been debated and they increase the risk of infection by providing a false sense of safety.

Expert opinion recommends the disinfection of the phlebotomy site by a appropriate antiseptic solution with a combination of alcohol and a long acting antiseptic to have an effective residual activity and good cleansing action for reducing the risk of blood contamination or bacteremia. Benzalkonium chloride synergized with ethanol is a highly effective broad spectrum antiseptic with quick contact times against bacteria, enveloped viruses, pathogenic fungi and mycobacteria.

## INJECTA™

- **INJECTA™** contains ethanol proven for quick antiseptic action.
- **INJECTA™** contains optimum concentration of ethanol (70% v/v IP) to ensure diffusion through the cell membrane of microbes, for effective antisepsis.
- **INJECTA™** contains 0.5% w/v benzalkonium chloride, a rapidly acting biocide with effective residual activity and cleansing action.
- The synergistic combination of benzalkonium chloride with ethanol in **INJECTA™** ensures bactericidal, virucidal and fungicidal activity with quick contact times.
- **INJECTA™** is produced under FDA compliant GMP.

## HAND DISINFECTION

Concept of hand hygiene emerged in the 19th century. Ignaz Semmelweis and Joseph Lister, introduced cleaning hands with antiseptics (1847) and antiseptic surgery (1867) respectively.

Early solutions contained chlorides of lime and soda for hand disinfection. 1961 saw the implementation of handwash training. Hand hygiene in the present scenario is achieved by:

- Washinghand using antimicrobial soap (with antiseptic property)
- Decontaminating hands with broad spectrum and quick drying hand rub.

**Handwashing** involves washing hands with plain soap (without antiseptic property) and water.

**Antiseptic handwash** involves mechanically removing dirt and loosely adherent transient flora from the hands, inactivating strongly adherent transient flora and part of resident skin flora with the help of antiseptic detergent (Figure 4.6).

**Alcohol-based handrub** involves disinfecting hands by rubbing them with an alcohol containing (no water) preparation for surgical hand hygiene/antisepsis before operations by surgical personnel.

As per the new Centers for Disease Control and Prevention (CDC), USA guidelines on Hand Hygiene (October, 2002) washing hands with antimicrobial soap and water is required when:

- Hands are visibly soiled (dirty)
- Hands are visibly contaminated with blood or body fluid
- Before eating
- After using the rest room.

### Hand Hygiene is Required

### *Before*

Contact with a patient, donning gloves, inserting urinary catheters, peripheral vascular catheters, or other invasive devices that do not require surgery and before surgery.

### *After*

Contact with a patient's skin, contact with body fluids or excretions, non-intact skin, wound dressings, removing gloves.

While selecting a right antiseptic for hand hygiene one must look for the:

- Efficacy of antiseptic agent
- Acceptance of product by healthcare personnel based on the characteristics of product, skin irritation and dryness of the skin

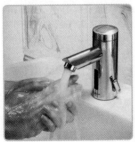

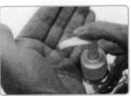

**Figure 4.6** Handwash

Handwash          Handrub

- Accessibility of product
- Dispenser systems.

### Handwash v/s Handrub

Handwashing may be sufficient in many (non-critical) situations during patient care but use of hygienic hand rubs provides a much higher level of safety with little time and effort.

STERIMAX® is an antiseptic handrub with triple action. It has synergistic power of 3 molecules – Alcohol + Chlorhexidine + Triclosan. STERIMAX® has long-lasting residual activity, is pleasantly perfumed with skin emollients, has broad spectrum antimicrobial activity, is resistance-free, is non-sticky and skin safe.

STERIMAX® is for use:
- Before entering clean room/sterile areas like OT, ICU, NICU
- In OT before surgery—just before putting on surgical gloves
- In OT after surgery—after handwashing
- Before and after handling patients in wards
- Before and after handling patients and babies at home
- Skin prepping before IV administration
- Preventing dermal infections
- Dressing of minor injuries
- First aid for cuts, bites, abrasions
- General purpose disinfection.

STERIMAX® is available in 100 mL, 500 mL and 5 L pack sizes.

### Environment and Surface Disinfection

The rise in the occurrence of various diseases is becoming a huge problem. Three most important components which play an important role for an infection to occur are—a susceptible host, a pathogenic microorganism and an environment that is congenial for the multiplication of the pathogen. Air and surfaces play very important role in transmission of infection.

Dust particles are reservoir for microorganism. Dust particles of 5 micron are able to remain suspended in air. Airborne infections are transmitted directly or indirectly through air. Similarly, contaminated surfaces pass on the infection to anyone coming in contact with it, e.g. mops and cleaning cloths get contaminated as they come in contact with a contaminated surface and transfer increasing number of microorganisms to subsequent surfaces they touch. Therefore, air and surface disinfection is necessary to reduce the infection rate by reducing the number of pathogens present in the environment.

Air in the absence of HEPA filters contains contaminants or pathogens. Air in the OT gets contaminated with each surgery. Movement in OT increases dust particle in suspension.

**Methods generally used for disinfection are:**
General disinfection by either of the following methods—

- Cleaning with carbolic acid and fumigation with formaldehyde
- Cleaning with aldehyde based germicides and fumigation with formaldehyde
- Cleaning floor with peroxygen compounds, instruments with aldehyde based germicides and fumigation with formaldehyde:

Disadvantages of these methods are:
- Time consuming: Minimum 24 hours turnover time required (carbolic acid + formaldehyde)
- Leaves sticky surface due to surfactant base (aldehydes)
- Have limited efficacy (carbolic acid + peroxygens)
- Efficacy neutralizes due to combination of oxidizing agent and reducing agent (peroxygens + aldehydes)
- Formaldehyde is highly irritant to skin, eye and nose
- Formaldehyde is a known carcinogen.
  AEROSEPT™ is a quick drying disinfectant spray for air and surfaces. It has powerful rapid broad spectrum biocidal and synergistic action. AEROSEPT™ is all surface compatible and non-corrosive. AEROSEPT™ is an effective antiviral including H1N1 and HIV.

AEROSEPT™ can be used:
- To rapidly disinfect surfaces in OT, NICU, ICU
- To rapidly disinfect NICU pumps, ECG monitors, ventilators, incubators, pulse oxymeters, monitors, fibrillators, respiration and AVD units, dental chairs, equipments, beds, table tops, etc.
- To rapidly disinfect airspace between patient and surgeries.

Apply liberally to the site being disinfected and mop the area using sterile cotton.

MICROLYSE® is a powerful disinfectant and cleaner for hard surfaces. It is broad spectrum disinfectant effective against bacteria, fungi and viruses (including H1N1 and HIV). Has instant and residual action. It is all surface compatible and non-corrosive. High use dilution of MICROLYSE® makes it cost-effective.

MICROLYSE® can be used as a daily disinfectant to disinfect hard surfaces in:
- OT, NICU, ICU, wards, OPD, clinics, pathology laboratories, blood banks
- Production and processing areas of food and drug industries, clean rooms/ sterile areas, R&D laboratories, QA/QC laboratories, corridors, toilets, etc.

## LABORATORY GLASSWARE CLEANING AND DISINFECTION

### LABCLENZ™

LABCLENZ™ is a laboratory cleaner for glasswares, equipments made of plastic, porcelain, ceramics, quartz and stainless steel. It is formulated to remove grease, smudges, fingerprints and grime on glass and surfaces.

Anionic and non-ionic surfactants in Labclenz remove both organic and inorganic materials and metal ions from laboratory equipments.

## Composition

Minimum 0.6 % sodium hypochlorite, non-Ionic and anionic surfactants, stabilizers.

## Directions for Use

- Use 2 % v/v solution of Labclenz in demineralized water (preferably warm) for washing applications
- Glass, plastics, quartz, porcelain and ferrous metal apparatus can be cleaned safely and effectively in 2 % v/v solution of Labclenz
- Spray on surface. Wipe or dry with a paper towel or cloth
- Labclenz is easily and completely eliminated by rinsing-preferably with distilled or demineralized water. It leaves no traces susceptible to interfere in further analyzes.

# Chapter Five

# Healthcare Facilities: Waste Management

The proper management of Health Care Facilities (HCF) waste depends on good administration and organization along with adequate legislation, financing and active participation of trained staff. HCF waste is a special type of waste carrying a high potential of infection and injury. Waste is generated in HCF refers to biological or non-biological that is discarded, and is not intended for further use in a hospital. According to a WHO report, around 85% of the hospital wastes are actually nonhazardous, 10% are infective (hence, hazardous), and the remaining 5% are non-infectious but hazardous (chemical), pharmaceutical and radioactive. Poor management of health care waste may expose health care personnel, waste handlers, and the community to infectious agents, toxic materials, and an increased risk of injury. It may have serious significant impact on the environment. The purpose of proper management of (HCF) waste management is:

- To eliminate the possibility of acquired infection through unauthorized, inappropriate access to clinical waste and to minimize adverse effects resulting from contact with waste pharmaceuticals.
- To satisfy concerns regarding the general standard of HCF's hygiene.

It is the responsibility of the HCF's management and all the staff and the Environmental Health Department Management.

The equipment needed for waste management in HCF's as the follow: Color coded puncture proof plastic containers, color coded plastic liners (bags) with a variety of sizes (big, medium and small) for collection of different types of infected and non-infected wastes, a sealing mechanism at the neck of the bag (tie), puncture protection gloves and waste collection trolleys (Figure 5.1).

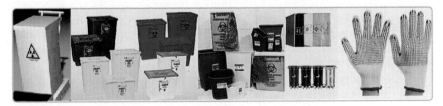

**Figure 5.1** Waste management implements

## WASTE CLASSIFICATIONS

HCF's wastes are divided into the following groups:

### Non-Medical Waste (or Non-Hazardous Waste)

General or non-medical waste poses no additional risk of injury or infection to staff, to patients, to visitors, or to the community at large. It is similar in composition to household trash.

### Medical Waste (Hazardous Waste)

Medical waste consists of several different sub-categories such as:

1. **Infectious waste**—includes all waste items that are contaminated with or suspected of being contaminated with body fluids (Blood and blood products, used catheters and gloves, cultures and stocks of infectious agents, waste from dialysis and dentistry units, from isolation units, wound dressings, nappies, discarded diagnostic samples, infected animals from laboratories, and contaminated materials (swabs, bandages, and gauze) and equipment (disposable medical devices, e.g. IV fluid lines and disposable spatulas).
2. **Anatomic wastes**—consist of body parts and tissues (e.g. placenta), waste from clinical laboratories and animal carcasses.
3. **Sharps waste**—consists of all of the following:
   - Needles, used and unused, unless still sealed in the original packaging
   - Syringes contaminated with biohazardous waste whether or not a needle is attached
   - Slides, blades
   - Root canal files; orthodontic wires
   - Acupuncture needles
   - Needles and syringes from a household when generated by a health care professional during a home visit
   - Broken glass items contaminated with biohazardous waste, thin walled unbroken glass contaminated with biohazardous waste such as capillary tubes or ampules
   - Any item capable of cutting or piercing that is contaminated with trauma scene waste.
4. **Chemical waste**—containing chemical substances e.g., laboratory chemicals, empty bottles of laboratory or pharmacy chemicals, disinfectants that have expired or are no longer needed, solvents, diagnostic kits, poisonous and corrosive materials, and cleaning agents and others.
5. **Pharmaceutical waste**—containing pharmaceutical substances include: expired, unused and contaminated pharmaceuticals, e.g. expired drugs, vaccines and seras.
6. **Genotoxic waste**—consists of highly hazardous, mutagenic, teratogenic, or carcinogenic waste containing substances with genotoxic properties, include: Cytotoxic, neoplastic drugs used in cancer treatment, their metabolites and genotoxic chemicals. See Table 5.1 for classification of hazardous medical waste.

**Table 5.1** Classification of hazardous medical waste

| | |
|---|---|
| 1. Sharps | 1. Waste entailing risk of injury |
| 2. Waste entailing risk of contamination | 2. Waste containing blood, secretions or excreta entailing a risk of contamination |
| 3. Anatomical waste | 3. Body parts, tissue entailing a risk of contamination |
| 4. Infectious waste | 4. Waste containing large quantities of material, substances or cultures entailing the risk of propagating infectious agents (cultures of infectious agents, waste from infectious patients placed in isolation wards) |
| 5. Pharmaceutical waste | 5. Spilled/unused medicines expired drugs and used medication receptacles |
| 6. Genotoxic waste | 6. Expired or leftover Genotoxic drugs, equipment contaminated with cytotoxic substances |
| 7. Chemical waste | 7. Waste containing chemical substances: Leftover laboratory solvents, disinfectants, photographic developers and fixers |
| 8. Radioactive waste | 8. Waste containing radioactive substances: Radionuclides used in laboratories or nuclear medicine, urine or excreta of patients treated. |

7. **Radioactive materials**—unused liquids from radiotherapy or laboratory research; contaminated glassware, packages, or absorbent paper; urine and excreta from patients treated or tested with radioactive substances.
8. **Miscellaneous waste**—including items such as bedding and laundry/ kitchen wastes.

## Biohazard Symbol

Biohazard presented as standard for all biological hazards since 1966 , it must be placed on biohazardous waste containers. The symbols investigated had to meet a number of criteria: (1) Striking in form in order to draw immediate attention; (2) Unique and unambiguous, in order not to be confused with symbols used for other purposes; (3) Quickly recognizable and easily recalled; (4) Easily stenciled; (5) Symmetrical, in order to appear identical from all angles of approach; and (6) Acceptable to groups of varying ethnic backgrounds." The chosen scored the best on nationwide testing for memorability. It is used in the labeling of biological materials that carry a significant health risk (Figure 5.2 biohazard symbols).

## Segregation and Color Coding of Clinical Waste

- **Segregation means** the separation of the entire waste generated in a hospital in defined, different waste groups according to the specific treatment and disposal requirements. Only a segregation system can ensure that the waste will be treated according to the hazards of the waste and that the correct disposal routes are taken and that the correct transportation equipment will be used.
- **Color coding means** to combine different waste groups with "similar" hazards in one main group and to identify this main group in a fast and easy way by a fixed color.

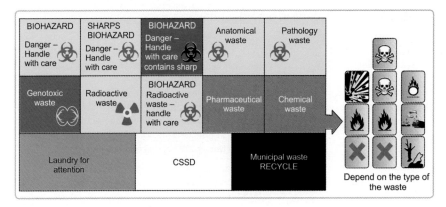

**Figure 5.2** Biohazard symbols

The simplest way to identify the different types of waste is to collect the various types of waste in separate containers or plastic bags that are color-coded and/or marked with a symbol as the following:

## Group A

Healthcare waste with similar composition to household and municipal waste:

### *Color Code*

Black

### *Packaging*

Black plastic bags of good quality.

### *Symbol*

None

*Profound segregation:* The national introduced colors for the to be recycled materials should be used, the international recycling sign should be placed on the bags.

## Group B

Biomedical and infectious healthcare waste.

### *Colour Code*

Yellow.

### *Packaging*

None-reusable puncture-proof container. If a separate collection of sharps in special sharp containers is introduced, plastic bags not less then 90 microns can be used for other infectious waste.

### Symbol

International biohazard symbol in black and wording "Biohazardous waste" and "Danger—Handle with Care—Contains Sharp Items"

## Group C

Sharps.

### Color Code

Yellow.

### Packaging

None-reusable puncture-proof container.

### Symbol

International biohazard symbol in black and wording "Biohazardous Waste" and "Danger—Handle with Care—Contains Sharp Items." Suitable container should be as the following:

- Puncture-resistant, leak-proof, shatter-proof and able to withstand heavy handling.
- Displays the universal biohazard label and has a label clearly indicating the nature of the contents.
- Has an opening which is accessible, safe to use, and designed so that it is obvious when the container is full.
- Is sealed when full or ready for disposal can be handled without danger of the contents spilling or falling out.

## Group D

**Microbiology and Biotechnology Waste** (Wastes from laboratory cultures, stocks or specimen of live microorganisms or attenuated vaccines, human and animal cell cultures used in research and infectious agents from research and industrial laboratories, wastes from production of biologicals, toxins and devices used for transfer of cultures).

### Color Code

Red.

### Packaging

None-reusable puncture-proof autoclavable container. If a separate collection of sharps in special sharp containers is introduced, plastic bags not less then 90 microns can be used for other infectious waste.

### Symbol

International biohazard symbol in black and wording "Biohazardous Waste" and "Danger—Handle with Care—Contains Sharp Items"

## Group E
Anatomical and pathological waste.

### Color Code
Yellow.

### Packaging
Water tight and sealable strong yellow plastic bags or containers.

### Symbol
International biohazard symbol in black and wording "Biohazardous Waste" "Incinerate Only" "Anatomical Waste", or human specimens or tissues that have been fixed in formaldehyde or other fixatives. Secondary containers must be labeled "Pathology Waste".

*Note:* Best-management practice is to store anatomical waste in the freezer.

## Group F
Genotoxic waste.

### Color Code
Purple.

### Packaging
Sealable, robust containers, appropriately for their content and for normal conditions of handling and transportation.

### Symbol
Cell in telophase, wording: "Genotoxic Waste"

## Group G
Radioactive waste.

### Color Code
Yellow.

### Packaging
Sealable, robust containers, appropriately for their content and for normal conditions of handling and transportation.

### Symbol
International radioactive symbol, wording: "Radioactive Waste"

## Group H
Chemical waste.

### Color Code
Brown.

### Packaging
Sealable, robust containers, appropriately for their content and for normal conditions of handling and transportation.

Hazardous chemical waste of different types should never be mixed.

### Symbol
Depend on the type of the waste, such as: oxides, corrosive, mixed hazards, environmental polluting materials, etc.

## Group I
Pharmaceutical waste.

### Color Code
Brown.

### Packaging
Sealable, robust containers, appropriately for their content and for normal conditions of handling and transportation.

### Symbol
Depend on the type of the waste.

## Group L
Laundry bag.

### Color Code
Blue.

### Packaging
Sealable, appropriately for their content and for normal conditions of handling and transportation.

### Symbol
None, wording: "Laundry for the attention".

### Group S

Instruments soiled with blood or body fluids.

### *Color Code*

Clear plastic

### *Packaging*

Sealable, appropriately for their content and for normal conditions of handling and transportation.

### *Symbol*

None, wording: "CSSD".

## MANAGEMENT OF REUSABLE INSTRUMENTS

### Handling

Medical waste should be handled as little as possible before disposal. It should not be collected from patient-care areas by emptying into open carts; this may lead to contamination of the surroundings and to scavenging of waste as well as to an increased risk of injury to staff, clients and visitors.

### Bag Filling

Waste and sharps containers should be discarded when they become three quarters full and at least once daily or after each shift. The reason for this is to reduce the risk of plastic bags splitting open and of an injury from a protruding sharp item in sharps containers.

### Medical Waste Labeling

Two opposite sides of the exterior of the package should be labeled clearly in lettering that is readable at a minimum distance of five feet as the following:
1. Word 'BIOHAZARD'.
2. Word 'Sharps' if the package contains sharps.
3. International Biohazard Symbol.

In addition, the generator must securely attach a water-resistant label or tag to each package and write in indelible ink:
1. Generator's name.
2. Generator's address.
3. Generator's phone number (24-hour number, if available).

The transporter must also affix a label to each package in the same manner:
1. Transporter's name.
2. Transporter's permit number.
3. Transporter's address.

4. Transporter's phone number (24-hour number, if available).
5. For each package, the date when waste initially left the generator's site, or a unique ID number giving that information.

## Medical Waste Storage

General waste may be stored in a separate room at the facility, pending collection by the contractor.

- All the waste (group B and D) must be stored in a designated area with access limited to authorized, personnel only, infectious waste should be disposed of within 24 hours.
- All laboratory waste (group E) shall be stored in a refrigerated, lockable, closed storage pending disposal.

## Interim Storage

Waste should be transported to interim storage at the end of every shift. To reduce the risk of infection and of injury, minimize the amount of time waste is stored at the facility. Waste should be stored in an area of controlled access that is minimally trafficked by staff, clients, and visitors. It is preferable to have a room to store waste on each floor of the facility, but, if this is difficult, one central storage room should be designated. The storage area should also be included in a cleaning schedule; interim storage time should not exceed two days.

## Interim Storage Area Requirements

- Contain medical waste in a manner that is not offensive and that minimizes the threat to health, safety or the environment.
- Store all containers of medical waste in a secure location.
- Ensure all necessary equipment required to clean and disinfect the area in case of accidental spillage is easily available and accessible.
- Treat any waste mixed with medical waste, as medical waste.
- Sharps such as needles, syringes with needles and surgical instruments should not incorporate cutting, bending or any other manipulation that could generate aerosols or splatter contaminated fluids.
- Place all medical waste other than sharps in clearly labelled heavy duty color coded plastic bags.
- Tie the bags so as to prevent leakage or expulsion of solid or liquid wastes during storage, handling or transport and ensure they will not be subject to compaction by any compacting device.
- There must be enough space around stored waste containers/ bags to allow regular inspection for leakage or label deterioration.
- Waste should not be stored close to patients or where food is prepared.

## Characteristics of Medical Waste Storage Areas at Health Care Facilities

- Storage areas should have an impermeable hard floor with good drainage that can be easily cleaned and disinfected.
- They should have a water supply for cleaning purposes.

- Storage areas should afford easy access for staff-in-charge of handling the waste.
- It should be possible to lock the storage area to prevent access by unauthorized persons.
- Easy access for waste collection vehicles is essential.
- Storage areas should be protected from the sun.
- Storage areas should be inaccessible to rodents, dogs, cats, insects, birds, and other animals.
- There should be good lighting and ventilation.
- Storage areas should not be situated in proximity of food storage or preparation areas.
- A supply of cleaning equipment, protective clothing, and waste bags or containers should be located conveniently close to the storage area for use by waste management staff.

## Medical Waste Collection

The internal waste management plan for the health care facility should stipulate regular procedures and schedules by which waste is collected daily or as frequently as required and transported to a designated central storage site which, more than likely, will be the contractor's point of collection. Various units will generate different types of medical waste as the following:

### Medical Wards

Infectious waste such as dressings, bandages, sticking plaster, gloves, disposable medical items, used hypodermic needles and intravenous sets, body fluids and excreta, contaminated packaging, and meal scraps.

### Operating Rooms and Surgical Wards

Anatomical waste such as tissues, organs, fetuses, and body parts as well as other infectious waste and sharps.

### Laboratories

Pathological (including some anatomical), highly infectious waste (small pieces of tissue, microbiological cultures, stocks of infectious agents, infected animal carcasses, blood and other body fluids), and sharps plus some radioactive and chemical waste. Urine may be carefully poured down the sewer.

### Pharmaceutical and Chemical Stores

Small quantities of pharmaceutical chemical waste consisting mainly of packaging, and general waste.

### Support Units

General waste comparable to municipal solid waste.

## General Waste Collection Requirements

- General non-medical waste should be handled within the health care facility's domestic refuse system.
- Sharps should all be collected together, regardless of whether or not they are contaminated. Sharps containers should be puncture-proof and usually are made of metal or high-density plastics. Sharps containers should be tamperproof and fitted with covers that do not allow access to the sharps contained within. The containers should be rigid and impermeable so that they safely retain not only the sharps but also residual liquids from syringes.
- Bags for infectious waste should be red and marked with the international infectious substance symbol.
- Bags and containers should be removed when they are no more than three quarters full to enhance their safe handling. Some bags can be closed by tying the neck of the bag while heavier gauge bags may require plastic sealing ties of the self-locking type.
- Cytotoxic waste should be collected in strong, leak proof containers that are clearly labeled as cytotoxic wastes.
- Large quantities of obsolete or expired pharmaceuticals stored at hospital wards or departments should be returned to the pharmacy for disposal.
- Large quantities of chemical waste should be placed in chemical resistant containers and sent to specialized treatment facilities if they are available. The identity of the chemicals should be clearly marked in the containers and hazardous chemical wastes of different types should not be mixed.
- Wastes with high content of heavy metals such as cadmium and mercury should be collected separately for disposal at appropriate locations.

## Medical Waste Transportation

The transport medical waste on-site from generation locations to the point of collection or storage, health care facilities must assure that this is done safely. This may require the use of wheeled trolleys, containers, or carts that are not used for any other purpose and must meet the following specifications:

- Easy to load and unload
- No sharp edges that could damage waste bags or containers during loading and unloading
- Easy to clean and disinfect at least daily

## Transport Vehicles and Containers

Waste bags may be placed directly into the transportation vehicle but it is usually safer to place them in additional containers such as a cardboard box or a wheeled, rigid, plastic, or galvanized bin. While this results in an advantage of reducing the handling of filled medical waste bags, it may also result in higher transportation costs. Any vehicle used to transport medical waste should have the following general design characteristics:

1. The body of the vehicle should be of a suitable size commensurate with the amount of medical waste that it must transport.

2. There should be a bulkhead between the driver's cab and the vehicle body designed to retain the load if the vehicle is involved in an accident.
3. All vehicles should be placarded on both sides and rear. The placard must be marked with relevant hazard symbol and word identifying the load. The symbol and words shall be bold and readable from at least 30 meters away.
4. There should be a suitable system for securing the load during transport.
5. Empty plastic bags, suitable protective clothing, cleaning equipment, tools, disinfectant, and special kits for dealing with liquid spills should be carried in a separate compartment in the vehicle.
6. The internal finish of the vehicle should allow it to be steam cleaned.
7. The internal angles of the waste storage compartment should be rounded for easier cleaning.
8. The vehicle should be marked with the name and address of the contractor.
9. The international biohazard sign should be displayed on the vehicle or container as well as an emergency telephone number.
10. Vehicles used for transporting medical waste should not be used for the transportation of any other material.
11. Vehicles should be kept locked at all times except when loading and unloading.
12. Two or more kinds of incompatible wastes shall not be loaded together in a single vehicle since it would be a risk of violent reaction or fire, generate a harmful gas, or render the materials more dangerous to deal with.

## Medical Waste Treatment

The choice of treatment and disposal techniques depends on a number of parameters: the quantity and type of wastes produced, whether or not there is a waste treatment site near the hospital, the cultural acceptance of treatment methods, the availability of reliable means of transport, whether there is enough space around the hospital, the availability of financial, material and human resources, the availability of a regular supply of electricity, whether or not there is national legislation on the subject, the climate, groundwater level, etc.

The method must be selected with a view to minimizing negative impacts on health and the environment. There is no universal solution for waste treatment. The option chosen can only be a compromise that depends on local circumstances. Where there is no appropriate treatment infrastructure in the vicinity, it is the responsibility of the hospital to treat or pre-treat its wastes on-site. This also has the advantage of avoiding the complications involved in the transport of hazardous substances.

The primary methods of treatment of medical waste are:
• Incineration
• Autoclaves
• Chemical disinfection with grinding
• Microwave
• Irradiation
• Encapsulation (or solidification) of sharps
• Burial: Sanitary landfills, trenches, pits.

For all of these treatment types, the treated waste can generally be disposed with general waste in a landfill, or in some cases discharged into the sewer system. In the past, treatment of medical waste was primarily performed on-site at hospitals in dedicated medical waste facilities. Over time, the expense and regulation of these facilities have prompted organizations to hire private companies to collect, treat, and dispose of medical waste, and the percentage of medical organizations who perform their own treatment and disposal is expected to drop.

To ensure that each treatment method provides the proper environment for the destruction of biologicals, test packages containing a microbiological spore test indicator are regularly used to test the effectiveness of the treatment methods. Microbiological spores are the most difficult of biologicals to destroy, so when the test package cannot be cultured after treatment, the waste is considered properly treated. In treatment methods where shredding or maceration is employed, the test package is inserted into the system after the shredding process to avoid physical destruction of the test package. The test package is then retrieved from the waste after treatment.

## Incineration Treatment

It is the controlled burning of the medical waste in a dedicated medical waste incinerator. The waste generally passes through the incinerator on a belt, and because most medical waste can be incinerated, the waste is not sorted or separated prior to treatment. Incineration has the benefit of reducing the volume of the waste, sterilizing the waste, and eliminating the need for pre-processing the waste before treatment. The resulting incinerated waste can be disposed of in traditional methods, such as brought to a landfill. The downside of incineration is potential pollution from emissions generated during incineration. The incineration process can be applied to almost all medical waste types, including pathological waste, and the process reduces the volume of the waste by up to 90%.

Modern incinerators can provide a secondary benefit by harnessing the heat created by the incineration process to power boilers in the facility. The flames in the primary chamber can ignite fossil fuels in a secondary chamber and power facility boilers.

The largest concern associated with incineration is pollution and the biggest concern is the incineration of chemicals that are released from combusting plastics. While incineration provides the advantage of reducing the volume of waste into ash and the ability to dispose recognizable waste and sharps, the incinerator may contain toxic gasses. Dioxins and furans can be produced when these plastics burn. The majority of older medical waste incinerators contain no pollution control equipment. As new federal and state emission regulations are instituted that have more stringent requirements, medical incinerators are often not being replaced at the end of their service life. Over time, the amount of waste being incinerated will be reduced as other technologies replace on-site incinerators. Another concern is related to the contents of incinerator ash. As incinerators are designed or retrofit with pollution prevention equipment, more of the potentially toxic chemicals that previously ended up in emissions now remain in the ash. Incinerator ash is generally disposed of in landfills, and little data is available on the effects of ash on the environment.

As additional requirements are added to the emissions for medical waste incinerators, the cost of incinerating medical waste increases, and alternative treatments have increased their market share.

- All recognizable human anatomical remains (except teeth).
- Human specimens or tissues that have been fixed in formaldehyde or other fixatives. Secondary containers must be labeled "Pathology Waste" or "PATH".
- Waste that is contaminated through contact with, or having previously contained, antineoplastic agents. Secondary containers must be labeled "Chemotherapy Waste" or "CHEMO".

## Autoclave Treatment

Autoclaves are closed chambers that apply both heat and pressure, and sometimes steam, over a period of time to sterilize medical equipment. Autoclaves are used to destroy all microorganisms that may be present in medical waste before disposal in a traditional landfill. The autoclave lowers the pressure within the chamber, which shortens the amount of time required to generate steam.

Medical waste that is subjected to an autoclave is often also subjected to a compaction process, such as shredding, after treatment so that it is no longer recognizable and cannot be re-used for other purposes. The compaction process reduces the volume of the treated waste significantly. After treatment and compaction, the treated waste can be combined with general waste and disposed of in traditional manners. Waste that is treated using an autoclave is still recognizable after treatment, and therefore must be shredded after treatment to allow for disposal with general waste. Autoclaves are not recommended for the treatment of pathological waste, due to the recognizability factor after treatment, and that pathological waste may contain low levels of radioactive material or cytotoxic compounds. The autoclave process can aerosolize chemicals present in the waste and depending on the design of the autoclave, these chemicals can be released into the air when the autoclave is opened.

Steam autoclave is used mostly for surgical instruments. This method is not well-suited for heat sensitive materials and instruments. Many surgical instruments are not designed to withstand prolonged heat and moisture of the steam sterilization process.

Autoclaves can be used to process up to 90% of medical waste, and are easily scaled to meet the needs of any medical organization. Small counter-top autoclaves are often used for sterilizing reusable medical instruments. Large autoclaves are used to treat large volumes of medical waste at once.

Autoclaves include steam heating, dry heating, chemical sterilization, or ultraviolet light. Steam autoclaves are far more common, using heated, vaporized water to kill pathogens. Dry heat autoclaves use dry heat to sterilize instruments. They are used in cases where heating is the preferred method of pathogen destruction, but moisture could damage the inserted instruments. Chemical sterilizers can be broken down into two major groups, cold sterilizers and gas autoclaves. These devices are used in situations where heating could damage sensitive instrumentation, including plastic and rubber devices, fiber optics, etc. They do require external venting systems to remove the chemical agents from the sterilizer. These fans or drain systems may be integral to the device, although some models can be connected into existing exhaust systems.

Cold sterilization autoclaves use a cold sterilization liquid to sterilize the contents. Cold sterilization liquids have been developed to enable sterilization or high-level disinfection.

Gas autoclaves use a vapor solution to sterilize its contents. Unlike the humid environment produced by conventional steam, the unsaturated chemical vapor method is a low-humidity process. No time-consuming drying phase is needed, because nothing ever gets wet. Gas autoclaves generally require less heat-up time, as well, which allows for greater instrument turnover. Common sterilizing agents include formaldehyde gas and ethylene oxide.

Ultraviolet autoclaves and sterilizers produce ultraviolet light exerting a lethal effect on unwanted disease causing organisms. They can destroy pathogens, bacteria, mold spores, yeast, protozoa, fungi and algae.

## Chemical Disinfection with Grinding Treatment

The use of chlorine bleach for cleaning and disinfecting is well-known and this method has been in use for many years. The mechanical/chemical disinfection process provides control and consistency to the disinfection process. The EPA identifies chemical disinfection as the most appropriate method to treat liquid medical waste. Chemical disinfection processes are often combined with grinding of medical waste before exposing it to a liquid chemical disinfectant to ensures sufficient exposure of the chemical agent to all parts of the waste and helps in easy disposal of any residues. The disinfectant is usually combined with a large amount of water to assist with the disinfection process and to cool the mechanical equipment in the shredding process. The resulting liquids are dropped into the sewer system; solid residues are disposed in landfills.

## Microwave Treatment

Microwave treatment of medical waste uses a thermal combustion method of treatment that requires the waste to be shredded and mixed with water. Waste is shredded and moistened with steam. The material is then microwaved in a treatment chamber and shredded, then ground in a particulizer. The water is used as a heat transfer medium to evenly heat all portions of the waste and sterilize the entire mass for disposal. Microwave treatment of medical waste is effective at eliminating many hazards but the Environmental protection agency (EPA) does not recommend using microwave technology to sterilize pathological waste products.

The microwave treatment process uses radiant energy to heat moisture in the waste effectively killing infectious agents through a combination of heat and pressure.

Many smaller medical facilities choose microwave treatment technology due in part to the affordability of the unit and the ease of use. Unfortunately, microwave treatment cannot be used for all types of medical waste. Volatile chemicals and large mass waste is not suitable for treatment in a microwave unit. Sterilization of waste is monitored using biological or chemical indicators which assure that the waste is safe for disposal. Proper segregation of waste streams assures that hazardous chemicals are not fed into the treatment chamber. This further reduces the chance of harmful emissions resulting from the microwave treatment process.

Microwave treatment is a cost-effective treatment method for the safe preparation and disposal of regulated medical waste. Treating medical waste in a microwave unit, when combined with shredding, reduces the final waste volume by as much as 60%. This results in reduced disposal and hauling costs which can save the average hospital or medical facility as much as 20% in overall costs.

### Irradiation Treament

A method used to sterilize medical equipment or waste is irradiation, generally through exposure of the waste to a cobalt source. The gamma radiation generated by the cobalt source inactivates all microbes that may be present in the waste. The treated waste shreds after irradiation, and then ships the waste to a cement kiln, where it is burned as fuel. The cost of developing a dedicated facility for this method is quite high, and therefore this method is not as widely used as other treatment methods at this time.

### Encapsulation Treatment

Encapsulation (or solidification) consists of containing a small number of hazardous items or materials in a mass of inert material. The purpose of the treatment is to prevent humans and the environment from any risk of contact.

Encapsulation involves filling containers with waste, adding an immobilizing material, and sealing the containers. The process uses either cubic boxes made of high-density polyethylene or metallic drums, which are three-quarters filled with sharps, chemical or pharmaceutical residues, or incinerator ash. The containers or boxes are then filled up with a medium such as plastic foam, bituminous sand, lime, cement mortar, or clay. Once the medium has dried, the containers are sealed and disposed of in a sanitary landfill or waste burial pit. The main advantage of the process is that it is very effective in reducing the risk of scavengers gaining access to the hazardous waste. Encapsulation of sharps is generally not considered to be a long-term solution. Encapsulation of sharps or unwanted vaccines could, however, be envisaged in temporary settings, such as camps or vaccination campaigns.

### Sanitary Landfill or Waste Burial Pit Treatment

The disposal of untreated health-care waste in an uncontrolled dump is not recommended and must only be used as a last resort. It can be disposed of in a sanitary landfill, subject to certain precautions: it is important that health-care waste be covered rapidly. One technique is to dig a trench down to the level where old municipal refuse (over three months old) has been buried and to immediately bury health-care waste that is discarded at this level under a 2-metre layer of fresh municipal refuse.

The following are the essential factors that must be taken into consideration in the design and use of a sanitary landfill:

- Access must be restricted and controlled.
- Competent staff must be available.

- Discarding areas must be planned.
- Bottom of the landfill must be waterproofed.
- Water table must be more than 2 metres below the bottom of the landfill.
- There must be no drinking water sources or wells in the vicinity of the site.
- Chemicals must not be disposed of on these sites.
- Waste must be covered daily and vectors (insects, rodents, etc.) must be controlled.
- Landfill must be equipped with a final cover to prevent rainwater infiltration.
- Leachates must be collected and treated.

Whenever a municipal landfill is being used, the water and habitat engineer must inspect the site before hazardous medical waste are discarded there.

## Medical Waste Disposal

### *Disposal of Liquid Medical Waste*

Liquid medical waste can be poured down a sink, drain, and flushable toilet. If none of these are available, in a pit.

- Always wear heavy utility gloves and shoes when handling or transporting liquid medical waste.
- Afterwards, wash both gloves and shoes.
- Consider where the sink, drain or toilet empties.
- Avoid splashing the waste on yourself, on others or on surfaces.
- After disposal rinse the sink, drain, or toilet to remove residual waste, being careful to avoid splashing.
- Clean the fixture with a disinfectant solution at the end of each day or more often if heavily soiled.
- Decontaminate the container that held the liquid medical waste by filling it with a 0.5% chlorine solution and leaving it for 10 minutes before washing.

## Disposal of Hazardous Chemical Waste

Disposing of cytotoxic and radioactive waste should be done in accordance with all local and national laws and regulations.

- Always wear heavy utility gloves and shoes when handling or transporting hazardous chemical waste.
- Wash both gloves and shoes if they become contaminated.
- Cleaning solutions and disinfectants should be handled as liquid medical waste.
- Rinse containers thoroughly with water.
- Wash glass containers with detergent and water.
- Do not reuse plastic containers.

## Disposal of Dental Waste

### *Amalgam*

These particles are a possible source of mercury in the sewer system. Store waste amalgam in a closed container that is labeled as hazardous waste and list the contents and the date. Used and empty amalgam capsules may be disposed of as solid waste since they are nonhazardous.

- Practitioners are encouraged to follow "best management practices" in the handling and disposal of dental amalgam to limit its potential environmental effects.
- Practitioners are advised to use precapsulated dental amalgam to reduce the risk of liquid mercury spill or clinic–environmental contamination.
- Alternative restorative materials (i.e., composite resin, ceramic or other metal alloys) can be used.
- Practitioners are legally responsible for the collection, storage and disposal of both gross debris and fine amalgam particles removed via high-volume suction.
- Dental amalgam scrap as well as amalgam waste gathered by filters and separation devices should be collected periodically and stored in a labeled, leak-proof container (e.g., in a dry mercury-vapor suppressant system).
- The proper storage of dental amalgam will also reduce the amount of elemental mercury vapor that enters the work environment.
- Contaminated wastewater should not be flushed down sinks, nor place material containing dental amalgam in general garbage or waste to be incinerated.

### Amalgam Separators

Separation technology is based on sedimentation, filtration or centrifugation of the dental amalgam particles from waste water. The proper amalgam separation unit must be selected carefully as not all units are able to work efficiently in every physical arrangement. Some units are placed before vacuum pumps, others after. Some require considerable space to house the unit, while others are compact.

#### Silver

Silver is another heavy metal that can enter water system via improper disposal of dental office waste. Although silver is a component of dental amalgam, the silver thiosulfate in radiographic fixer presents a greater environmental concern. Some forms of silver are more toxic than others; for example, silver thiosulfate is less toxic than free silver ions. Used radiographic fixer must not be washed down the drain. The best way to manage silver waste is through recovery and recycling. Dentists can install in-house silver recovery units to salvage the silver themselves, allowing for some monetary return on the equipment investment when the silver is later sold. These units generally recover silver ions from the waste solution through displacement of iron ions or through a closed-loop electrolytic system that recovers not only silver for reuse, but also the radiographic fixer. Alternatively, the waste can be collected by a registered agency certified to carry and manage the waste.

### Dental Unused Film

It should not be placed in the general waste; unused films contain unreacted silver that can be toxic in the environment. Safe disposal can generally be accomplished by simply contacting the supplier of the product and returning the waste for recycling. Alternatively, a certified waste carrier can be contacted to dispose of the waste, ideally by recycling. With recent advances in radiographic technology, digital imaging is becoming a popular means of obtaining dental radiographs. Among its advantages are reduced radiation exposure and the absence of chemical image processing. Therefore, incorporation of digital imaging within the dental office can greatly reduce the amount of silver waste generated.

## Lead

An additional by-product of traditional radiography is the lead shields contained in each film packet. Although the lead shields themselves are relatively small, the cumulative waste produced can be considerable. An added benefit of digital radiography is the reduction in lead waste production. Lead, like mercury and silver, is toxic and persists in the environment. Even at low levels of exposure, lead exerts adverse health effects on both children and adults. The lead shields from film packets merely have to be collected and returned periodically to the manufacturer for recycling. The only cost is for postage. Unfortunately, some manufacturing companies report that only about 5% of products sold are returned. In part, it appears that this is due to a lack of awareness of the offered service.

## Dental Used X-ray Fixer

Collect and store used fixer in a closed plastic container labeled with the words, "Hazardous Waste-Used Fixer," and the date that the fixer was first added. When enough fixer has accumulated (usually 5–10 gallons), a recycling service contactor should pick-up the used fixer. Fixer and developer should not be mixed together. The other option for disposing of used X-ray fixer is to install a silver recovery unit at the end of the X-ray processing unit. The recovered silver can be sold to a metal reclaimer, and the treated fixer can be disposed of down a drain. However if there is a connection to a septic system, fixer cannot be dispose down a drain.

## Dental X-ray Film

Silver can be reclaimed from X-ray film. Reclamation companies that accept used fixer will often take X-ray film as well. Label the container as hazardous waste.

## Lead Foil

Reclamation companies that accept used fixer also may accept lead foil. Another possible outlet for recycling lead foil is through your dental supply company. Label the container as hazardous waste.

## Developer

Used developer can be disposed of down a drain (sewered) that is connected to a publicly owned treatment works.

## Cleaners for Developer Systems

If cleaners contain chromium, they must be manifested and disposed of as hazardous waste. It may be easier and cheaper to use cleaners that do not contain chromium.

### Traps and Filters

First, disinfect a disposable trap by soaking it for 24 hours in a minimum amount of disinfectant. Then, remove all visible amalgam and store it in a dry, covered container. Wear a mask and gloves during this process. The disinfected trap then should be autoclaved and disposed of as solid waste. If it is not autoclaved, it must be disposed of as infectious waste.

### Reusable Traps

Like the disposable traps, first disinfect a reusable trap by soaking it for 24 hours in a minimum amount of disinfectant. Then remove all visible amalgam and store it in a dry, covered container. Wear a mask and gloves during this process. The disinfected trap then should be autoclaved. After autoclaving, dispose of the contents as solid waste and reuse the trap.

### Used Linen Managment

Put all linen soiled with blood or body secretions, in isolation bag then in blue laundry bag marked "laundry for the attention".

### Management of Reusable Instruments

All instruments soiled with blood or body fluids should be put first in isolation bag and then in clear plastic bag marked "CSSD". In small facilities where CSSD does not exist a clear decontamination and sterilization policy should be developed in accordance with infection control principles and strictly adhered to.

## STAFF PROTECTION MEASURES

The handling of waste entails health risks for staff throughout the chain. The purpose of protective measures is to reduce the risks of accident/exposure or the consequences. Preventive measures can be divided into two categories as following:

### Primary Prevention

- Eliminating hazard: For example, by using less toxic substances, eliminating mercury, or using self-locking injection equipment.
- Collective and technical prevention: For example, using needle receptacles, ventilation.
- Organizational prevention: Such as assigning duties and responsibilities to all involved, management (sorting, packaging, labelling, storage, transport), best practices (such as refraining from putting the caps back on syringes), training.
- Individual prevention: Personal protective equipment, vaccination, washing hands (Tables 5.2 and 5.3).

### Secondary Prevention

- Measures in the event of an accident (accidental exposure to blood, spills).

■ **Table 5.2** Personal protective equipment (PPE)

| | |
|---|---|
| Face protection—face shield Eye protection—safety goggles | To be worn during all activities where body fluids or chemicals are liable to be splashed, and for work at an incinerator |
| Respiratory protection—masks and respirators | FFP1 dust respirators23 for staff involved in any activity that generates dust (removing ash, sweeping out the waste storage facility) FFP2 respirators24 for staff involved in handling waste from patients suffering, for example, from tuberculosis • FFP1-FFP2-FFP3 dust respirators do not provide protection from gas and fumes (such as mercury or solvent fumes) • Surgical masks protect the patient; they provide only limited protection for staff |
| Body protection—aprons, protective suits | For staff involved in collecting, transporting and treating wastes |
| Hand protection—gloves | Disposable gloves for care staff or cleaning staff (vinylor nitrile) Disposable gloves for laboratory staff (nitrile). Heavy-duty protective gloves for staff involved in transporting and treating wastes • Latex gloves are to be avoided (can cause allergy) • Nitrile is more chemical-resistant and tear-resistant than vinyl |
| Foot and leg protection—boots, shoes | Closed, non-slip shoes for all staff. Puncture-proof safety shoes or boots |

## Personal Hygiene

Elementary personal hygiene is important for reducing risks of infections and breaking the infection chain when medical waste is being handled. Ideally, wash basins with hot water and soap should be installed wherever wastes are handled (storage and treatment areas).Washing one's hands meticulously with a sufficient amount of water and soap eliminate over 90 % of the microorganisms present.

## Handwash

- When going on and off duty
- After any contact with wastes
- After removing gloves
- After removing a mask or respirator
- Before/after certain routine actions (eating, using the toilet, blowing one's nose)
- Wet the hands and wrists
- Apply a dose of liquid soap
- Lather the soap by rubbing the hands, paying particular attention to the parts between the fingers and around the nails and to the thumbs (40–60 seconds)

**Table 5.3** Risks of infection associated with hazardous medical waste

| Type of infection | Infective agent | Transmission agent |
| --- | --- | --- |
| Gastrointestinal infections | Enterobacteria (Salmonella, *Vibrio cholerae*, Shigella, etc.) | Feces, vomit |
| Respiratory infections | *Mycobacterium tuberculosis, Streptococcus pneumoniae,* SARS virus (Severe acute respiratory syndrome), Measles virus | Inhaled secretions, saliva |
| Eye infections | Herpes virus | Eye secretions |
| Skin infections | Streptococcus | Pus |
| Anthrax | *Bacillus anthracis* | Skin secretions |
| Meningitis | *Neisseria meningitidis* | Cerebrospinal fluid |
| AIDS | Human immunodeficiency virus (HIV) | Blood, sexual secretions, other body fluids |
| Hemorrhagic fever | Lassa, Ebola, Marburg, and Junin viruses | Blood and secretions |
| Viral hepatitis A | Hepatitis A virus | Feces |
| Viral hepatitis B and C | Hepatitis B and C viruses | Blood and other biological fluids |
| Avian influenza | H5N1 virus | Blood, feces |

- Rinse
- Dab dry
- Do not use a brush (which promotes the penetration of microorganisms).
- Risks of Infection associated with hazardous medical waste are listed in Table 5.3.

## Vaccination

The hepatitis B virus disease can be avoided by vaccination, which has been available since 1980. Numerous studies have shown that the vaccine is effective in preventing all of the forms of infection with hepatitis B virus. Although this vaccination is safe, effective and cost-efficient, it is still underused.

Staff handling wastes must be appropriately protected by vaccination, including vaccination against hepatitis A and B and tetanus (Table 5.3).

# Bibliography

1.  APIC Guidelines Committee. Association for Professionals in Infection Control and Epidemiology, INC. Am J Infec Contr. 1996;24:313–42.
2.  Ascenzi JM. Handbook of disinfectants and antiseptics. New York, Marcel Dekker; 1996.
3.  Bartz JC, Kincaid AE, Bessen RA. Rapid prion neuroinvasion following tongue infection. Journal of Virology. 2003;77:583–91.
4.  Bellinger-Kawahara C, et al. Purified scrapie prions resist inactivation by UV irradiation. J Virol. 1987;61:159–66.
5.  Berg P, et al. Asilomar conference on recombinant DNA molecules. Science. 1975; 188:991–94.
6.  Biological safety cabinets—biological safety cabinets (Class I) for personnel and environment protection. Sydney, Standards Australia International, 1994 (Standard AS 2252.1–1994).
7.  Biological safety cabinets—laminar flow biological safety cabinets (Class II) for personnel, environment and product protection. Sydney, Standards Australia International, 1994.
8.  Biosafety in microbiological and biomedical laboratories. 4th ed. Washington, DC, United States Department of Health and Human Services/Centers for Disease Control and Prevention/National Institutes of Health, 1999.
9.  Block SS. Disinfection, sterilization and preservation. 5th ed. Philadelphia, Pennsylvania, Lippincott Williams & Wilkins, 2001.
10. Bosque PJ, et al. Prions in skeletal muscle. Proceedings of the National Academy of Sciences of the United States of America. 2002;99:3812–17.
11. Centers for Disease Control and Prevention. Recommendations for prevention of HIV transmission in health-care settings. Morbidity and Mortality Weekly Report. 1987;36 (2):1S–18S.
12. Collins CH, Kennedy DA. Laboratory acquired infections: history, incidence, causes and prevention. 4th ed. Oxford, Butterworth-Heinemann; 1999.
13. Furr AK. CRC handbook of laboratory safety. 5th ed. Boca Raton, FL, CRC Press, 2000.
14. Garner JS. Hospital infection control practices advisory committee. Guideline for isolation precautions in hospitals. Am J Infect Contr. 1996; 24:24–52,
15. Glatzel M, et al. Extraneural pathologic prion protein in sporadic Creutzfeld-Jakob disease. NEJM. 2003; 349:1812–20.
16. Health Canada. Laboratory biosafety manual. 2nd ed. Ottawa, Minister of Supply and Services, Canada; 1996.
17. Health Services Advisory Committee. Safe working and the prevention of infection in clinical laboratories. London, HSE Books; 1991.
18. Hunt GJ, Tabachnick WJ. Handling small arbovirus vectors safely during biosafety level 3 containment: Culicoides variipennis sonorensis (Diptera: Ceratopogonidae) and exotic blue- tongue viruses. JME. 1996;33:271–7.

19. Infection control guidelines for hand washing, cleaning, disinfection and sterilization in health care. 2nd ed. Ottawa, Laboratory Centre for Disease Control, Health, Canada; 1998.

20. Infectious substances shipping guidelines. Montreal, International Air Transport Association, 2003 (http://www.iata.org/ads/issg.htm).

21. Laboratory Biosafety manual. Geneva, World Health Organization. 3rd ed. 2004.

22. Lewis RJ. Sax's dangerous properties of industrial materials. 10th ed. Toronto, John Wiley and Sons; 1999.

23. National Research Council. Occupational health and safety in the care and use of research animals. Washington, DC, National Academy Press, 1997.

24. O' Malley BW Jr, et al. Limitations of adenovirus-mediated interleukin-2 gene therapy for oral cancer. Laryngoscope. 1999; 109:389–95.

25. Richmond JY, Quimby F. Considerations for working safely with infectious disease agents in research animals. In: Zak O, Sande MA, (eds). Handbook of animal models of infection. London, Academic Press, 1999;69–74.

26. Russell AD, Hugo WB, Ayliffe GAJ. Disinfection, preservation and sterilization. 3rd ed. Oxford, Blackwell Scientific; 1999.

27. Rutala WA. APIC guideline for selection and use of disinfectants. 1994, 1995, and 1996.

28. Safar J, et al. Prions. In: Richmond JY, McKinney RW, (eds) Biosafety in microbiological and biomedical laboratories. 4th ed. Washington, DC, United States Department of Health and Human Services. 1999;134–43.

29. Safety in health-care laboratories. Geneva, World Health Organization. 1997, (http://whqlibdoc.who.int/hq/1997/WHO_LAB_97.1.pdf ).

30. Sattar SA, Springthorpe VS, Rochon M. A product based on accelerated and stabilized hydrogen peroxide: evidence for broad-spectrum germicidal activity. CJI Cont. 1998;13:123–30.

31. Schneider PM. Emerging low temperature sterilization technologies. In: Rutala WA (ed). Disinfection and sterilization in health care. Champlain, New York, Polyscience, 1997;79–92.

32. Springthorpe VS, Sattar SA. Chemical disinfection of virus-contaminated surfaces. CRC Critical Reviews in Environmental Control. 1990;20:169–229.

33. Springthorpe VS. New chemical germicides. In: Rutala WA (ed). Disinfection and sterilization in health care. Champlain, New York, Polyscience, 1997;273–80.

34. Standards Australia/Standards New Zealand. Biological safety cabinets— installation and use. Sydney, Standards Australia International, 2000.

35. Taylor DM, et al. The effect of formic acid on BSE and scrapie infectivity in fixed and unfixed brain-tissue. Veterinary Microbiology, 1997;58:167–74.

36. Technical instructions for the safe transport of dangerous goods by air, 2003–2004 Edition. Montreal, International Civil Aviation Organization, 2002.

37. Thomzig A, et al. Widespread PrPSc accumulation in muscles of hamsters orally infected with scrapie. EMBO Reports. 2003;4:530–33.

38. Transport of Infectious Substances. Geneva, World Health Organization, 2004.

39. A Study of Hospital Waste Management System in Command Hospital (Southern Command), Pune. A dissertation submitted to University of Pune. WG CDR RK Ranyal, Dec 2001; p. 37.

40. Acharya DB, Singh M. The book of hospital waste management. Minerva Press, New Delhi. 2000;15:47.

41. Anderson K. Creating an environmentally friendly dental practice. CDS Rev. 1999; pp. 12–8.
42. Baldwin, CL, Runkle, RS. "Biohazards symbol: development of a biological hazards warning signal." Oct 13 Science. 1967;158 (3798): 264–5.
43. Chin G, Chong A, Kluczewska A, Lau A, Gorjy S, Tennant M. The environmental effects of dental amalgam. Aust Dent J. 2000; 45(4):246–9.
44. Daughton CG. Cradle-to-cradle stewardship of drugs for minimizing their environmental disposition while promoting human health. II. Drug disposal, waste reduction, and future directions. Environ Health Perspect. 2003;111(5):775–85.
45. Government of India, Ministry of Environment and Forests Gazette Notification No. 460 dated July 27, New Delhi. 1998;10–20
46. Blenkharn JI. Standards of clinical waste management in UK hospitals. Journal of Hospital Infection. 2006;62 (3): 300-3.
47. Jones DW. Putting dental mercury pollution into perspective. Br Dent J. 2004; 197(4):175–7.
48. Kolpin DW, Furlong ET, Meyer MY, et al. Pharmaceuticals, hormones, and other organic wastewater contaminants in U.S. streams, 1999–2000: a national reconnaissance. Environ Sci Technol. 2002;36(6):1202–11.
49. National AIDS Control Organization. Manual of Hospital infection control. New Delhi. 1998; 50-66.
50. Park K. Hospital Waste Management. Park's textbook of preventive and social medicine. M/s Banarasidas Bhanot Publications, New Delhi. 18th Edn. 2005;595-98.
51. Razdan P, Singh A Cheema. Bio-medical waste management system. Proceedings of ASCNT–2009, CDAC, Noida, India. pp. 26 – 31.
52. Rao SKM, Garg RK. A study of hospital waste disposal system in service hospital. J Acad Hosp Admini. July 1994; 6(2):27-31.
53. Singh IB, Sarma RK. Hospital waste disposal system and technology. J Acad Hosp Admini. July 1996;8(2):44-8.
54. Srivastava JN. Hospital Waste Management Project at Command Hospital. Air Force, Bangalore. National Seminar on Hospital waste Management: A report. 27 May 2000.
55. Singh VP, Biswas G, Sharma JJ. Biomedical waste management—An Emerging Concern in Indian Hospitals. 2007–07 to 2007–12) Vol. 1, No. 1 (.http://www.indmedica.com/journals.php?journalid=11&issueid=98&articleid=1324&action=article.
56. www.absa.org/abj/abj/000502Turnberg.
57. www.icrc.org/spa/assets/files/.../icrc-002-4032.
58. www.searchmedica.co.uk/search.html.

# Index

Page numbers followed by *f* refer to figure and *t* refer to table